W0081259

Chakra Organized Acceptance and Commitment Therapy

This book integrates the traditional chakra model, which provides a map-like tool for how psycho-emotional content interacts with the physical body, with current evidence-based psychological practice.

As growing research highlights the impact of psychosocial trauma on physical health and the prevalence of medically unexplained symptoms, novel treatment approaches are required to address the unique complexities of these conditions. Drawing from humanistic psychology and Acceptance and Commitment Therapy (ACT), this book presents a holistic model for treating psychosomatic disorders. Chapters focus on the basic principles of the chakra system, treatment orientation, and key areas of intervention: developing body awareness, self-integration, and values-based action.

This book is an essential introduction to working with the chakra system in the context of behavioral health interventions and is suitable for all healthcare professionals, in particular clinical psychologists, therapists, and counselors.

Rosemary Hale (PsyD) is a clinical psychologist and life-long learner and advocate for integrative health practices. She works as a primary care behavioral consultant in Indiana, USA, where she specializes in guiding patients towards health behavior change and values-based actions to promote mental and physical wellness.

Chakra Organized Acceptance and Commitment Therapy

Treating Psychosomatic Conditions

Rosemary Hale

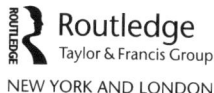

Routledge
Taylor & Francis Group

NEW YORK AND LONDON

Designed cover image: Getty Images

First published 2023
by Routledge
605 Third Avenue, New York, NY 10158

and by Routledge
4 Park Square, Milton Park, Abingdon, Oxon OX14 4RN

Routledge is an imprint of the Taylor & Francis Group, an informa business

Library of Congress Cataloging-in-Publication Data
A catalog record for this title has been requested

ISBN: 978-1-032-16986-6 (hbk)
ISBN: 978-1-032-16982-8 (pbk)
ISBN: 978-1-003-25129-3 (ebk)

DOI: 10.4324/9781003251293

Typeset in Garamond
by Taylor & Francis Books

To my grandmothers, Rosemary and Luanna. You have taught me more than I could ever express, including to believe in myself and follow my own path. And to my girl, Sydney, the light of my life.

Contents

Illustrations

Figures

Tables

Preface

This work is the blending of several passions and lessons from different phases of my life. At each point, it was the teachers, supervisors, and healers I met along the way who shaped my ideas and guided me towards the clinician I would eventually become. I was fascinated with mind-body medicine at a young age, partially due to my own experience navigating a chronic and medically-unexplained vertigo. Multiple rounds of physical therapy, vestibular therapy, and psychotherapy helped me understand the psychosomatic processes influencing my symptoms. I also began taking classes on Eastern religion and philosophy as I was exploring my own existential beliefs. In college, I learned about the field of health psychology, and found my intellectual home. I was also given the opportunity to study mindfulness-based therapies and self-discrepancy theory at the University of Oxford before completing my undergraduate degree in psychology from Oglethorpe University. The conversations I had with my Oxford tutors laid the groundwork for the work in this book. The spring/summer before I entered my doctorate program, I picked up Caroline Myss's *Anatomy of the Spirit*[1] and began my discovery of the chakras. I was immediately captivated by a system that illustrated such details of the mind-body-spirit connection. I entered my doctorate program with the intention of creating a self-report measure of the chakras, a tool that could be used within health psychology and transpersonal studies. With the support of my dissertation chair and committee, I was lucky enough to enjoy the process of completing my doctoral project, and my interest in this work continued to grow. I was fortunate again during my predoctoral internship year to have mentors that encouraged my passions as I dived into the world of Acceptance and Commitment Therapy (ACT). It was like finding the missing piece. The theory behind ACT aligned with much of what I had been exploring personally and professionally during my key developmental years. By the end of my internship year, I had started writing this book. The ideas presented in this book reflect who and where I am today, the culmination of a journey through and to myself. I humbly hope that this work may help to guide others in their own self journey.

With gratitude,

Rosemary

Note

1 Myss, C. (1996). *Anatomy of the Spirit*. Three Rivers Press.

Acknowledgements

My love and thanks to my husband Kyle, who patiently listened as I talked through many ideas and helped review each chapter. I am also incredibly thankful for the professors, teachers, and supervisors that helped me develop into the clinician and person I am today. A special mention to Drs Nicole Taylor, Lisa Elwood, Jaqueline Hess, Matthew Grant, Sarah Dross-Gonzalez, Jackie Maxwell, Leah Zinner, John Carton, Margaret Yee, and Alla Yankouskaya. I must acknowledge those who developed Acceptance and Commitment Therapy (ACT/FACT), particularly Steven C. Hayes, Kirk Strosahl, and Patricia Robinson. Their influence is surely evident in how often they are cited throughout this book. My appreciation also to David Clarke, whose work introduced me to the study of psychophysiologic disorders. Lastly, to my parents and all the friends and family that have encouraged my passions and always believed I could do anything I set my mind to.

Introduction

Psychosomatic Conditions

In the last two decades, mind-body medicine has been a rapidly-growing area of research and clinical focus. Mind-body medicine has brought attention to centralized chronic pain and psychosomatic conditions, also termed medically-unexplained symptoms or "functional somatic syndromes" (Bakal et al., 2008). "Centralized" pain refers to conditions where factors other than level of inflammation or tissue damage predict the severity of pain reported. These conditions demonstrate that subjective reports of pain and functional impairment often do not correlate with structural or tissue damage, but rather with psychological distress. Several studies have demonstrated that objective measures (e.g., MRIs) of organ disease or structural abnormalities are not reliable predictors of persistent pain/discomfort, and abnormal findings are common even among asymptomatic populations (Frank et al., 2015; Girish et al., 2011). Further, individuals with negative affective states tend to report more physical symptoms (Costa & McCrae, 1987), even in the presence of no objective health differences (Williams et al., 2002). One study found that 63 percent of asymptomatic subjects had minor disc herniations comparable to those in symptomatic subjects, and that psychological factors (e.g. stress) best discriminated between symptomatic and asymptomatic disc herniation (Boos et al., 1995). The fact that psychological and environmental factors influence subjective reports of pain is consistent with findings from social psychology (e.g., Schacter & Singer, 1962) and biofeedback research (e.g., Valins, 1967). People tend to rely on environmental information to interpret cues from the body, and then report physiologic, cognitive, and emotional experiences that match their understanding of the context.

Somatic symptoms are common even among healthy individuals, and include dizziness, chest pain, and shortness of breath. The majority of individuals with somatic symptoms will only seek medical treatment, and may be resistant to learning that psychological factors may be more relevant than any organic cause for their symptoms. Follow-up studies on patients with benign chest pain found that many patients who were told

DOI: 10.4324/9781003251293-1

they did not have a heart problem continued to engage in illness behaviors (e.g., restricting activity, scheduling medical appointments, emotional distress due to symptoms) (Bass, 1992). Clinical research has demonstrated that higher rates of somatization are associated with psychological distress, particularly anxiety and depression (Simon & Vonkorff, 1991). Further, psychosomatic symptoms may be due to atypical sensations or mis-interpretations of normal physiological processes (Bakal, 1999). The pain, and associated distress, is equally valid regardless and requires appropriate treatment.

Pain

Chronic pain is the most reported and studied psychosomatic symptom, as pain is the main reason people seek medical treatment (CDC, 2010). Health economists have estimated the cost of pain in the United States is over six billion dollars annually (Gaskin & Richard, 2012). A 2018 CDC report estimated that 11 to 40 percent of U.S adults experience chronic pain, which is associated with reduced mobility, opioid use and dependence, anxiety and depression, poor self-perceptions of health, and lower quality of life (Dahlhamer et al., 2018). In the 1990s there was a push for physicians to treat pain as a "fifth vital sign", in an attempt to better meet the large need for pain treatment in the US population. However, most treatments consisted of merely pain medication with a goal to eliminate or reduce pain. There was little discussion about coping with pain, improving psychosocial functioning, or maintaining physical activity, and the use of opioid medi-cations soared. The US is still combatting an opioid crisis, and many Americans continue to be dependent on pain medication, despite reporting ongoing pain symptoms.

Chronic pain is defined as pain that persists beyond three months; however, pain often lasts years or even decades. Pain also persists without structural cause or beyond the healing of any anatomical damage that occurred. When acute pain due to illness or injury becomes chronic, it is hypothesized that pain becomes learned through the repeated activation of the same neural pathways even after the injury has healed. Chronic pain is often conceptualized as a sensory disorder of the central nervous system, which can be comorbid with structural or tissue damage, as in the case of rheumatic conditions (e.g., lupus, gout, rheumatoid arthritis). However, even these conditions demonstrate components of centralized pain, meaning that subjective pain correlates with factors other than inflammation and tissue damage.

While pain normally serves as an important warning that the body is being harmed, this system malfunctions in the case of chronic pain. Acute pain instructs one to move their body out of harm's way, rest an injury, or otherwise engage in behaviors that promote healing. Chronic pain alerts the brain to the same actions, but when no threat is present. Individuals then make behavioral changes, such as limiting mobility or activity, but their pain does not improve. Often, the pain worsens due to the body weakening from lack of activity. Although the pain may not be caused by underlying structural damage, the pain experience of the patient is no less real or significant. Healthcare providers need to understand these differences in etiology and symptom processes in order to provide effective treatment. Treating chronic pain the same as acute pain with immobility and pain medication is largely ineffective for pain reduction, and counterproductive through deteriorating physical and psychosocial health.

Chronic pain appears to be connected with memory and emotional networks in the brain. Increased rates of chronic pain are associated with greater neural connectivity between the nucleus accumbens and prefrontal cortex (Baliki et al., 2012), which are both involved in emotional processing. Further, emotional distress is both a cause and consequence of physical pain. Functional brain scans show that patients with chronic pain display greater activity in emotional processing parts of the brain, while those with acute pain have higher activity in somatosensory areas (Hashmi et al., 2013). Interestingly, emotional pain activates the same areas of the brain as nociceptive pain (Kross et al., 2011), and recalling a painful emotional event can increase muscle tension associated with physical pain (Quartana & Burns, 2007). The fact that emotional and physical pain are processed similarly in the brain can make it difficult for individuals to accurately identify the cause of their pain, and difficult for healthcare providers to treat. An individual may not be aware that the source of their pain is emotional, and focusing on physical pain may be negatively reinforced by the avoidance of emotional pain (Lane et al., 2018). Failing to accurately identify the pain causes frustration for both the provider and patient as treatments are ineffective and the patient continues to experience somatic distress.

Historically, pain treatment has relied on a biomedical model which seeks to identify the cause of pain and eliminate it. Within this model, pain is believed to be a symptom of some underlying condition. This approach is often effective for acute episodes of pain, but works poorly for chronic pain. Today, treatment for chronic pain has shifted towards a biopsychosocial model (Engel, 1997). This model views pain as a condition in its own right, and includes an assessment of the various life factors known to influence pain (e.g., physical activity, emotional distress, pain beliefs, stress, coping skills, medication use, social support). Treatment focuses on modifying these factors to improve functioning and quality of life, rather than seeking to eliminate pain. The biopsychosocial model encourages a more holistic view of each individual and the context of their pain. This "whole health" approach emphasizes evidence-based strategies that can improve health in various domains (e.g., physical, emotional, social, spiritual).

Pain vs. Suffering

It is important to distinguish between pain and suffering. Pain is unavoidable. Pain is the body's natural and helpful response to a harmful or dangerous experience. Without pain, individuals would not remove their hand from the hot stove or run away from someone threatening them. Alternatively, suffering is emotional distress in response to current or anticipated pain. Suffering occurs when a person is dissatisfied with their present, past, or expected future situation and believes no action can resolve this discrepancy (Fordyce, 1995). When individuals experience suffering, distress about pain becomes the primary issue, rather than pain itself (Bakal, 1999). Unlike pain, suffering is not a necessary part of life. One way of reducing suffering is to respond to pain with awareness, understanding, and acceptance. This attitude towards pain is an example of psychological flexibility, the key change mechanism of Acceptance and Commitment Therapy or ACT (Hayes, Stroshal, & Wilson, 2012). ACT is an evidence-based treatment for chronic pain and focuses on improving functioning rather than eliminating pain. The ACT framework is presented throughout this text.

Trauma and Psychosomatic Symptoms

The seminal work of Felitti and colleagues (1998) on adverse childhood experiences (ACEs) initiated a scientific interest regarding the impact of stressful life events on physical health. The study found that the degree of household dysfunction and exposure to abuse during childhood increases one's risk of developing many leading causes of death and disability in adulthood. Individuals with four or more ACEs have more negative health outcomes throughout the lifespan (Bellis et al., 2013), and have been found to be twice as likely as those with no ACEs to develop painful conditions (Sachs-Ericsson et al., 2017). There is a dose-response relationship, meaning that greater ACEs are associated with increased risk of serious medical conditions, such as heart disease, cancer, lung disease, diabetes, autoimmune conditions, obesity, and chronic pain (Kalmakis & Chandler, 2015). ACEs also increase the risk of psychological dysfunctions including substance use, suicidality, posttraumatic stress disorder (PTSD), depression, and anxiety (Rhee et al., 2019). Social support and close relationships, alternatively, are important protective factors that improve recovery from ACEs (Brewin et al., 2000).

Many researchers have replicated and expanded on the findings of the original ACEs study (e.g., Davis et al., 2005). Afari and colleagues (2014) found that those exposed to trauma were nearly three times more likely to develop a functional somatic syndrome (e.g., chronic fatigue, irritable bowel syndrome, fibromyalgia). Another study found the prevalence of PTSD in chronic pain populations was four times the general population prevalence (Akhtar et al., 2019). PTSD has also demonstrated a high comorbidity with various "ill-defined" or "medically unexplained symptoms" in the cardiovascular, respiratory, musculoskeletal, neurological, gastrointestinal and immune systems (Gupta, 2013). Further, multiple forms of pain and trauma symptoms have often been found to co-occur and mutually maintain or exacerbate the other (e.g., Asmundson et al., 2002). For example, studies have found that individuals with chronic fatigue syndrome (CFS) are more likely to report post-traumatic stress symptoms (Krzeczkowska et al., 2015), and that a PTSD diagnosis may be associated with more severe CFS symptoms (Taylor et al., 2003). Sexual abuse and PTSD are also key risk factors for chronic pelvic pain (Meltzer-Brody et al., 2007).

Stress and the Body

Trauma experiences often lead to experiential avoidance strategies, or pushing away memories, thoughts, or feelings about the traumatic experience. However, "out of mind" does not mean "out of body" (Bakal, 1999). Even without conscious awareness of emotional pain, this distress can be expressed through somatic symptoms. Psychological stress is associated with a variety of negative health outcomes caused by changes in both the body and health behaviors; with stress-related healthcare costs estimated at $300 billion annually. Further, approximately three out of four people in the United States regularly experience physical symptoms (77 percent) and psychological symptoms (73 percent) caused by stress (American Institute for Stress, 2019).

At the nervous system level, stress activates the sympathetic nervous system, also called the "fight-or-flight" response. This system engages physiologic functions to energize and prepare the body for dealing with a threat, and signals changes throughout the body. The sympathetic nervous system operates through activation of the endocrine system, specifically the hypothalamus-pituitary-adrenal (HPA) axis which produces glucocorticoids (steroid hormones) including cortisol (the "stress hormone"). Cortisol helps regulate the immune system and inflammation in order to help the body cope with stress. This is designed to be a short-term response that ends once danger has passed. Long-term release of cortisol can negatively impact hormonal and immune system functioning, and contribute to developing conditions like chronic fatigue, diabetes, hypertension, hyperlipidemia, cardiovascular disease, obesity, depression, and anxiety (Maier et al., 1994). Chronic cortisol release is also associated with increased risk of infection due its immunosuppressant effect.

Within the reproductive system, cortisol impacts sexual functioning, as well as factors related to conception. Stress tends to reduce the sexual drive, and can contribute to reduced testosterone and erectile dysfunction in men. Stress also affects sperm production, maturation, mobility, and morphology. In women, stress can alter the length, regularity, and symptoms associated with the menstrual cycle. Women may experience greater pain or mood symptoms during menstruation, or miss cycles. Stress can make it more difficult for a woman to get pregnant, and negatively impact the health of both her and the child. Stress can also increase the risk of reproductive infection in men and women (e.g., herpes simplex complex), or exacerbate existing conditions (e.g., polycystic ovarian syndrome in women).

In the gastrointestinal system, stress alters gut bacteria which impacts mood. Stress can also prompt individuals to eat less/more and consume foods higher in sugar or carbohydrates. Further, increased alcohol or tobacco/nicotine use is associated with stress, and can increase heartburn and acid reflux. Stress can lead to difficulty swallowing due to spasms in the esophagus or ingesting large amounts of air when swallowing, causing burping and bloating. Individuals may experience pain or nausea in the stomach associated with stress. Stress can additionally affect the rate at which food is processed through the body, causing diarrhea or constipation, and how nutrients are absorbed into the body.

In the cardiovascular system, activation of the fight-or-flight response increases the heart rate, signals the heart to produce stronger contractions, and dilates blood vessels to increase blood flow. If prolonged, this increases the risk of hypertension, heart attack, and stroke. In the respiratory system, stress can cause shortness of breath or rapid breathing (e.g. hyperventilation), especially in those with pre-existing respiratory conditions such as asthma or chronic obstructive pulmonary disease (COPD). Lastly, stress increases muscle tension throughout the body. Muscles tighten in order to protect the body against pain or injury during acute stress, and then release when stress passes. Chronic stress leads to chronic tension, which leads to pain and the development of stress-related musculoskeletal disorders. Tension and migraine headaches, for example, are associated with tension in the shoulders, neck, and head (American Psychological Association, 2018).

Other Impacts of Trauma

There may be a genetic component in how trauma impacts the activation of certain genes. Genetic predispositions for a negative stress response and environmental experiences of trauma may interact to produce health problems later in life. In particular, experiences of adversity, poor social support, and lack of nurturance decrease effective coping with stress and disease resistance (Yanh et al., 2013). Unfortunately, familial patterns often demonstrate how trauma begets trauma through genetic and environmental conditions. For example, an individual who has experienced childhood abuse is more likely to be disconnected from their body's warning systems. As a result, they are also more likely to engage in experiential avoidance strategies, such as alcohol abuse or overeating, and more likely to be in an abusive relationship as an adult. Their child may then be genetically predisposed for a heightened stress response, and is also less likely to be in a supportive and nurturing environment due to the parent's own psychological distress and maladaptive coping style. These patterns of trauma and avoidance create the perfect storm for many mental and physical health problems to develop (Hayes, 2019).

Even subclinical levels of psychological distress, such as experiences of frustration, tension, and sadness, have been linked to negative health outcomes. Nonclinical negative alterations in mood and perceptions of social rejection reduce immune system functioning and increase pain sensitivity (Eisenberger et al., 2006). Hostility, for example, has been associated with increased risk of atherosclerosis as well as mortality due to any cause (Iribarren et al., 2000). Positive mood states and social support have the opposite effects (Bakal, 1999).

Somatic Symptoms of Psychological Distress

Symptoms of depression and anxiety are often associated with stressful or traumatizing experiences and can further manifest somatically. Older adults are especially vulnerable to somatization (Hegeman et al., 2012). Common physical symptoms of anxiety are muscle tension/aches, sleep disturbances, sweating, nausea and gastrointestinal discomfort, headaches, and an exaggerated startle response. Anxiety activates the sympathetic nervous system, which can cause accelerated heart rate, shortness of breath, dizziness, chest pain, feelings of choking, chills/heat, and numbing sensations. Physical symptoms of depression include fatigue, insomnia/hypersomnia, weight/appetite loss or gain, and psychomotor agitation or retardation; while many individuals additionally report body aches and pains (American Psychiatric Association, 2013). Patients often only seek medical care for these physical symptoms (Simon et al., 1999). Multiple physical symptoms of anxiety and depression are negatively associated with treatment outcomes (e.g., Huijbregts et al., 2010). Both anxiety and depression are further related to greater functional impairment in patients with medical diagnoses, including fibromyalgia, arthritis, and inflammatory bowel disease (Hirsch & Sirois, 2016).

Patients do not need to report psychological distress for their physical symptoms to be influenced by psychological factors. Medical providers may assume that patients who present with chest pain or dizziness but without subjective anxiety, do not have a psychosomatic component to their symptom. However, some individuals may experience less emotional distress because they experience their emotions somatically rather than cognitively. This may be unconscious or conscious efforts at emotional control (Bakal, 1999). Trauma and cultural experiences may also contribute to limited body and emotional awareness. Therefore, a psychosomatic condition may be present in the absence of reported emotional distress.

Context of Psychosomatic Conditions

Cultural context influences experiences of stress and pain. In the United States and in many other industrialized countries, individuals struggle against the societal norms that promote a fast-paced, work-dominated, individualistic, and materialistic way of life. In the pursuit of more success, money, recognition, etc., many feel intense pressure and high levels of stress. With all these daily demands, it is hard to imagine how anyone finds the time or energy to focus on their health and wellness. Conversations about self-care are increasing, but many still view self-care as luxury they cannot afford. Unfortunately, these patterns perpetuate a survival-mode or auto-pilot way of living, in which a sense of purpose and vitality is lost (Hayes, 2019). Individuals become disconnected from their body, self, relationships, and ultimately their life as they simply go through the motions of living without really experiencing life. These habits wreak havoc on one's health, while practicing adequate self-care (e.g., diet, exercise, sleep, relaxation, fun, and stress management) can improve both mental and physical health.

The treatment approach outlined in this book emphasizes tapping into an individual's own internal resources for self-healing. However, this requires an honest recognition of social and environmental factors outside an individual's control that impact health. It is more difficult to break the trauma response pattern when one is also facing any number of additional systemic social issues. On top of the increased risk for mental and physical health problems associated with trauma, many individuals are challenged with affordability and access barriers to basic living essentials (e.g. food, housing), education, healthcare, employment, and childcare, to name just a few. Add on issues of racism, discrimination, and prejudice, and it seems impossibly unfair to suggest individuals could heal themselves in such a context. Exposure to racial discrimination, for example, has been hypothesized as an explanation for the higher prevalence of hypertension in the United States Black population compared to other racial groups (Krieger & Sidney, 1996). Advocacy for social change is an important adjunct to the individual healing journey, and essential for minimizing and preventing the impact of trauma on health at both the individual and societal level.

Gender and Cultural Differences in Somatization

Somatization occurs cross-culturally, and there is a shared hesitancy to accept psychological explanations for symptoms (Janca et al., 1995). The most common somatic symptoms reported globally are sleep disturbances, muscle tension, headaches, back pain, and indigestion (Janca et al., 1995). An examination of World Health Organization (WHO) data from four-teen countries found that somatic symptoms are associated with emotional distress in both males and females. Females tend to report more somatic symptoms at each level of emotional distress. However, there was no difference in the number of somatic symptoms reported across cultures between males and females when emotional distress was controlled. The data also showed that more somatic symptoms were reported in less developed parts of the world (Piccinelli & Simon, 1997).

In the United States there is inconclusive and limited data regarding racial/ethnic variation in reports of somatization. It has been reported that African Americans and Hispanic/Latino Americans are more likely to report somatic symptoms of depression than White Americans (Lara-Cinisomo et al., 2020). However, another study found Latinx and Black Americans were no more likely to experience somatic symptoms of depression than their White counterparts (Sauceda et al., 2021). In a primary care setting, White and Latino Americans reported similar levels of physical symptoms, while Asian Americans reported significantly fewer. Greater acculturation in both Latino and Asian Americans was associated with increased physical symptoms (Bauer et al., 2012). While data is limited, it may be that exposure to trauma and/or adverse experiences better predicts somatization than race or ethnicity.

Primary Care

Psychosomatic conditions are especially prominent in primary care. Approximately one in three primary care visits are prompted by physical symptoms that receive a diagnosis of "medically unexplained," with 20–25 percent of these conditions becoming chronic (Kroenke, 2014). Lifetime prevalence rates in the general population are around 25 percent for many of the most common somatic symptoms, such as chest pain, back pain, dizziness, headache, and abdominal pain. A study of the ten most frequent physical complaints in primary care found that 85 percent of these patients had no diagnosable organic etiology, and patient satisfaction or improvement was generally below 50 percent at follow-up (Kroenke & Mangelsdorff, 1989). An analysis of the diagnoses received by patients who presented to primary care for symptoms with no organic etiology found that the most common diagnoses given were pain and somatization (25 percent), depression (20 percent), anxiety and panic (20 percent), job stress (10 percent), and marital and family problems (10 percent) (Tulkin & Gordon, 1998). Importantly, biopsychosocial evaluations that include an assessment for trauma can lead to a 35 percent reduction in primary care visits (Felitti & Anda, 2010).

Treatment of Psychosomatic Conditions

Many studies have demonstrated the efficacy of psychotherapeutic techniques for physical conditions (Abbass et al., 2008; Laird et al., 2016; Lumley et al., 2017). Behavioral treatments often include components of psychoeducation, relaxation training, cognitive restructuring, problem-solving, pain/symptom acceptance, exposure with reduced avoidance or safety behaviors, and values-based action (Riehl & Taft, 2021). Emotional Awareness and Expression

Therapy (EAET; Lumley & Schubiner 2019a) and Pain Reprocessing Therapy (Lumley & Schubiner 2019b) have more recently been established and supported as treatments specifically for psychophysiological disorders. These therapies focus on pain education, safety re-appraisal (reduce perceived danger of pain), and emotional processing (e.g., disclosure, writing, enactments, rescripting).

Integrative Medicine

Conventional medicine excels in the treatment of certain conditions, and largely fails in the treatment of others. For many, there is a desperate need for an alternative approach to healthcare that promotes general health and wellness while minimizing the risk of side effects. Physical, mental, emotional, and spiritual health are widely interconnected and to disregard one of these aspects does a great disservice to one's healing. Integrative medicine represents a functional and non-reductionist approach to health care that views health as more than merely the absence of disease, but instead as physical, mental, emotional, sociological, and spiritual wellbeing. The emphasis is on understanding the whole person in their context and utilizing the relationship between the care provider and the patient to enhance treatment outcomes.

Western philosophy and medical approaches tend to separate the mind from the body, such that the vast majority of health care providers are trained to work with either the physical body or the psychological mind, but rarely both. Health care providers tend to conceptualize a patient's symptoms only from the framework of their specialty. In the medical field, this means a patient with chronic migraines is likely to endure several unsuccessful medication trials and be referred for various expensive tests, scans, and consults before being asked about their stress levels or emotional functioning. In behavioral health, a therapist may spend several sessions trying to help a patient identify the thoughts and feelings that seem to trigger their anxiety, and miss that the patient is experiencing shortness of breath due to untreated asthma. Even worse, these providers often do not communicate even while treating the same individual for the same problem. Important information and opportunities for healing are missed when healthcare providers attempt to compartmentalize the human experience this way.

The immense gap left by biomedical approaches has led to an increasing interest in revisiting ancient medicine systems, particularly of Eastern traditions. Growing reliance on pharmaceuticals has disconnected people from the bio-intelligence of the body and its capacity for self-healing as individuals are treated for their symptoms without a functional understanding of their condition, Health providers wishing to adopt a more holistic approach must be willing to recognize the healing potential already within their patients, and view their role as encouraging this innate power (Bakal, 1999).

Providers must also allow their patients to be an equal partner in their healthcare treatment.

As psychosomatic conditions reflect biological, psychological, and social health-related factors, it follows that treatment should also integrate these domains (Singh, 2006). Yoga treatment approaches do just that, and have been studied with positive therapeutic effects for both physical and psychological conditions (Goyeche, 1979; Khalsa, 2004). Some of the most popular traditions of yoga include hatha (physical yoga), bhakti (devotional yoga), karma (service or action yoga), jnana (philosophical yoga), and raja (meditational yoga). Further, the chakra system, which originated with ancient yoga, offers a unique model for mapping how the physical, psychological, and spiritual aspects of an individual's experience overlap and influence one another.

From a yoga perspective, disease and illness is conceptualized as an energetic imbalance, and restoring energetic flow is thought to cure or resolve the problem. There are many ways that energy can be blocked, weakened, or entangled. Physical tensions (e.g., muscle tightness) can disrupt the flow of energy, but also mental tensions (e.g. fears, anxieties); both are manifestations of "wasted" energy (Rama et al., 1976). These energetic "black holes" only further consume valuable energy as many individuals seek, either consciously or unconsciously, to keep these painful experiences outside their awareness.

To better understand what helps people heal, 33 individuals were interviewed who had lived for several years after receiving a cancer diagnosis with a twenty percent or less probability of surviving five years (Berland, 1995). Five primary recovery attributions emerged: support of family and friends, attitudinal changes, medical treatment, spirituality, and alternative treatments. Twenty-eight reported that the key to their healing was a re-evaluation of their values and meaningful aspects of life. Over half of the participants believed that an existential change in how they perceived life was an important part of their healing. They reported improving their self-care habits (physically, psychologically, and spiritually), finding meaning and purpose in something larger than themselves, and committing to actions that fulfilled their newly uncovered true self and values. The treatment approach described in this book seeks to emulate these same monumental shifts – a change in how the patient relates to their body, self, and life.

References

Abbass, A., Lovas, D., & Purdy A. (2008). Direct diagnosis and management of emotional factors in chronic headache patients. *Cephalalgia*, 28(12), 1305–1314.

Afari N., Ahumada, S. M., Wright, L. J., Mostoufi, S., Golnari, G., Reis, V., & Cuneo, J. G. (2014). Psychological trauma and functional somatic syndromes: A systematic review and meta-analysis. *Psychosomatic Medicine*, 76(1), 2–11.

Akhtar, E., Ballew, A. T., Orr, W. N., Mayorga, A., & Khan, T. (2019). The prevalence of PTSD symptoms in chronic pain patients in a tertiary care setting: A cross-sectional study. *Psychosomatics*, 60(3), 255–262.

American Institute for Stress (2019, December 19). What is stress? Retrieved February 8, 2022, from https://www.stress.org/daily-life.

American Psychiatric Association. (2013). *Diagnostic and statistical manual of mental disorders* (5th ed.). Arlington, VA: American Psychiatric Publishing.

American Psychological Association. (2018, November 1). Stress effects on the body. http://www.apa.org/topics/stress/body.

Asmundson, G.J.G., Coons, M.J., Taylor, S., & Katz, J. (2002). PTSD and the experience of pain: Research and clinical implications of shared vulnerability and mutual maintenance models. *Canadian Journal of Psychiatry*, 47, 930–937.

Bakal, D. (1999). *Minding the body: Clinical uses of somatic awareness*. Guilford.

Bakal, D., Coll, P., & Schaefer, J. (2008). Somatic awareness in the clinical care of patients with body distress symptoms. *BioPsychoSocial Medicine*. 2(1), 6.

Baliki, M. N., Petre, B., Torbey, S., Herrmann, K. M., Huang, L., Schnitzer, T. J., Fields, H. L., & Apkarian, A. V. (2012). Corticostriatal functional connectivity predicts transition to chronic back pain. *Nature Neuroscience*, 15, 1117–1119.

Bauer, A. M., Chen, C. N., & Alegría, M. (2012). Prevalence of physical symptoms and their association with race/ethnicity and acculturation in the United States. *General hospital psychiatry*, 34(4), 323–331.

Bass, C. (1992). Chest pain and breathlessness: Relationship to psychiatric illness. *American Journal of Medicine*, 92(Suppl. 1A), 12–17.

Bellis, M.A., Lowey, H., Leckenby, N., Hughes, K. & Harrison, D. (2013). Adverse childhood experiences: Retrospective study to determine their impact on adult health behavior and health outcomes in a UK population. *Journal of Public Health*, 36(1), 81–91.

Berland, W. (1995). Unexpected cancer recovery: Why patients believe they survive. *Advances*, 11, 5–19.

Boos, N., Rieder, R., Schade, V., Spratt, K. F., Semmer, N., & Aebi, M. (1995). The diagnostic accuracy of magnetic resonance imaging, work perception, and psychosocial factors in identifying symptomatic disc herniations. *Spine*, 20, 2613–2625.

Brewin, C. R., Andrews, B., & Valentine, J. D. (2000). Meta-analysis of risk factors for posttraumatic stress disorder in trauma-exposed adults. *Journal of Consulting and Clinical Psychology*, 68(5), 748–766.

CDC (Centers for Disease Control and Prevention) (2010). Summary health statistics for U.S. adults: National health interview survey, 2009. Retrieved from http://www.cdc.gov/nchs/data/series/sr_10/sr10_249.pdf.

Costa, P. T., Jr., & McCrae, R. R. (1987). Neuroticism, somatic complaints, and disease: Is the bark worse than the bite? *Journal of Personality*, 55, 299–316.

Dahlhamer, J., Lucas, J., Zelaya, C., Nahin, R., Mackey, S., DeBar, L., Kerns, R., Vonkorff, M., Porter, L., & Helmick, C. (2018). Prevalence of chronic pain and high-impact chronic pain among adults- United States, 2016. *Center for Disease Control and Prevention, Morbidity and Mortality Weekly Report*, 67 (No. 36), 1001–1006.

Davis, D. A., Leucken, L., & Zautra, A. J. (2005). Are reports of childhood abuse related to the experience of chronic pain in adulthood? A meta-analytic review of the literature. *Clinical Journal of Pain*, 21(5), 398–405.

Eisenberger, N. I., Jarcho, J. M., Liberman, M. D., & Naliboff, B. D. (2006). An experimental study of shared sensitivity to physical pain and social rejection. *PAIN* 126, 132–138.

Engel, G. L. (1997). From biomedical to biopsychosocial: Being scientific in the human domain. *Psychotherapy and Psychosomatics*, 66, 57–62.

Felitti, V. J., & Anda, R. F. (2010). The relationship of adverse childhood experiences to adult medical disease, psychiatric disorders, and sexual behavior: Implications for healthcare. In R. Lanius & E. Vermetten (Eds.), *The Hidden Epidemic: The Impact of Early Life Trauma on Health and Disease* (pp. 77–87). Cambridge University Press.

Felitti, V. J., Anda, R. F., Nordenberg, D., Williamson, D. F., Spitz, A. M., Edwards, V., Koss, M. P., & Marks, J. S. (1998) Relationship of childhood abuse and household dysfunction to many of the leading causes of death in adults. The adverse childhood experiences (ACE) study. *American Journal of Preventive Medicine*, 14(4), 245–258.

Frank, J. D., Harris, J. M., Erickson, B. J., Slikker, W., Bush-Joseph, C. A., Salata, M. J., & Nho, S. J. (2015). Prevalence of femoroacetabular impingement imaging findings in asymptomatic volunteers: A systematic review. *Arthroscopy*, 31(6), 1199–1204.

Fordyce, W. E. (1995). What is pain? In W. E. Fordyce (Ed.), *Back pain in the workplace* (pp. 11–17). IASP Press.

Gaskin, D. J., & Richard, P. (2012). The economic costs of pain in the United States. *The Journal of Pain*, 13(8), 715–724.

Girish, G., Lobo, L. C., Jacobson, J. A., Morag, Y., Miller, B., & Jamadar, D. A. (2011). Ultrasound of the shoulder: Asymptomatic findings in men. *American Journal of Roentgenology*, 197(4), 713–719.

Goyeche, M. (1979). Yoga as therapy in psychosomatic medicine. *Psychotherapy and Psychosomatics*, 31, 373–381.

Gupta, M. A. (2013). Review of somatic symptoms in posttraumatic stress disorder. *International Review of Psychiatry*, 25, 86–99.

Hashmi, J. A., Baliki, M. N., Huang, L., Baria, A. T., Torbey, S., Hermann, K. M., Schnitzer, T. J., & Apkarian, A. V. (2013). Shape shifting pain: Chronification of back pain shifts in brain representation from nociceptive to emotional circuits. *Brain*, 136, 2751–2768.

Hayes, S. C. (2019). *A liberated mind: How to pivot toward what matters.* Avery.

Hayes, S. C., Strosahl, K. D., & Wilson, K. G. (2012). *Acceptance and commitment therapy: The process and practice of mindful change* (2nd ed.). Guilford.

Hegeman, J. M., Kok, R. M., van der Mast, R. C., & Giltay, E. J. (2012). Phenomenology of depression in older compared with younger adults: meta-analysis. *British Journal of Psychiatry*, 200, 275–281.

Hirsch, J. K., & Sirois, F. M. (2016). Hope and fatigue in chronic illness: The role of perceived stress. *Journal of Health Psychology*, 21(4), 451–456.

Huijbregts, K. M. L., van Marwijk, H. W. J., de Jong, F. J., Schreuders, B., Beekman, A. T. F., van der Feltz-Cornelis, C. M. (2010). Adverse effects of multiple physical symptoms on the course of depressive and anxiety symptoms in primary care. *Psychotherapy and Psychosomatics*, 79, 389–391.

Iribarren, C., Sidney, S., Bild, D. E., et al. (2000). Association of hostility with coronary artery classification in young adults. *JAMA*, 283, 2546–2551.

Janca, A., Isaac, M., Bennett, L. A., & Tacchini, G. (1995). Somatoform disorders in different cultures: A mail questionnaire survey. *Social Psychiatry and Psychiatric Epidemiology*, 30, 44–48.

Kalmakis, K. A., & Chandler, G. E. (2015). Health consequences of adverse childhood experiences: a systematic review. *Journal of the American Association of Nurse Practitioners*, 27(8), 457–465.

Khalsa, S. B. S. (2004). Yoga as a therapeutic intervention: A bibliometric analysis of published research studies. *Indian Journal of Physiology and Pharmacology*, 48(3), 269–285.

Krieger, N., & Sidney, S. (1996). Racial discrimination and blood pressure: The CARDIA study of young black and white adults. *American Journal of Public Health*, 86, 1370–1378.

Kroenke, K., & Mangelsdorff, A. D. (1989). Common symptoms in ambulatory care: Incidence, evaluation, therapy, and outcome. *American Journal of Medicine*, 86, 262–266.

Kroenke, K. (2014). A practical and evidence-based approach to common symptoms: A narrative review. *Annals of Internal Medicine*, 161(8), 579–586.

Kross, Berman, Mischel, Smith, & Wager. (2011). Social rejection shares somatosensory representations with physical pain. *Proceedings of the National Academy of Sciences of the USA*, 108, 6270–6275.

Krzeczkowska, A., Karatzias, T., & Dickson, A. (2015). Pain in people with chronic fatigue syndrome/myalgic encephalomyelitis: The role of traumatic stress and coping strategies. *Psychology, Health, & Medicine*, 20(2), 210–216.

Laird, K. T., Tanner-Smith, E. E., Russell, A. C., Hollon, S. D., & Walker, L. (2016). Short- and long-term efficacy of psychological therapies for irritable bowel syndrome: A systematic review and meta-analysis. *Clinical Gastroenterology and Hepatology*, 14(7), 937–947.

Lane, R.D., Anderson, F.S., & Smith, R. (2018). Biased competition favoring physical over emotional pain: A possible explanation for the link between early adversity and chronic pain. *Psychosomatic Medicine*, 80(9), 880–890.

Lara-Cinisomo, S., Akinbode, T. D., & Wood, J. A. (2020). Systematic review of somatic symptoms in women with depression or depressive symptoms: Do race or ethnicity matter? *Journal of Women's Health*, 29(10), 1273–1282.

Löwe, B., Spitzer, R.L., Williams, J. B. W., Mussell, M., Schellberg, D., & Kroenke, K. (2008) Depression, anxiety and somatization in primary care: Syndrome overlap and functional impairment. *General Hospital Psychiatry*, 30, 191–199.

Lumley, M.A. & Schubiner, H. (2019a). Emotional awareness and expression therapy for chronic pain: Rationale, principles and techniques, evidence, and critical review. *Current Rheumatology Reports*, 21(7), 30.

Lumley, M.A. & Schubiner, H. (2019b). Psychological therapy for centralized pain: An integrative assessment and treatment model. *Psychosomatic Medicine*, 81, 114–124.

Lumley, M.A., Schubiner, H., Lockhart, N. A., Kidwell, K. M., Harte, S. E., Clauw, D. J., & Williams, D. A. (2017). Emotional awareness and expression therapy, cognitive behavioral therapy, and education for fibromyalgia: A cluster randomized controlled trial. *Pain*, 158(12), 2354–2363.

Maier, S. F., Watkins, L. R., & Fleshner, M. (1994). Psychoneuroimmunology. The interface between behavior, brain, and immunity. *American Psychologist*, 49, 1004–1017.

Meltzer-Brody, S., Leserman, J., Zolnoun, D., Steege, J., Green, E., & Teich, A. (2007). Trauma and posttraumatic stress disorder in women With chronic pelvic pain. *Obstetrics & Gynecology*, 109, 902–908.

Piccinelli, M., & Simon, G. (1997). Gender and cross-cultural differences in somatic symptoms associated with emotional distress: An international study in primary care. *Psychological Medicine*, 27, 433–444.

Quartana, P. J., & Burns, J. W. (2007). Painful consequences of anger suppression. *Emotion*, 7, 400–414.

Rama, S., Ballentine, R., & Ajaya, S. (1976). *Yoga and psychotherapy: The evolution of consciousness*. Himalayan Publishers.

Rhee, T. G., Barry, L. C., Kuchel, G. A., Steffens, D. C., & Wilkinson, S. T. (2019). Associations of adverse childhood experiences with past-year DSM-5 psychiatric and substance use disorders in older adults. *Journal of the American Geriatrics Society*, 67(10), 2085–2093.

Riehl, M. E., & Taft, T. H. (2021). Working with patients with chronic digestive diseases. *Journal of Health Service Psychology*, 47(2), 97–104.

Sachs-Ericsson, N.J., Sheffler, J.L, Stanley, I. H., Piazza, J. R., & Preacher, K. J. (2017). When emotional pain becomes physical: Adverse childhood experiences, pain, and the role of mood and anxiety disorders. *Journal of Clinical Psychology*, 73(10), 1403–1428.

Sauceda, J. A., Patel, A. R., Santiago-Rodriguez, E. I., Garcia, D., & Lechuga. J. (2021). Testing for differences in the reporting of somatic symptoms of depression in racial/ethnic minorities. *Health Education & Behavior*, 48(3), 260–264.

Schacter, S., & Singer, J. E. (1962). Cognitive, social, and physiological determinants of emotional state. *Psychological Review*, 69, 379–399.

Simon, G. E, & Vonkorff, M. (1991). Somatization and psychiatric disorders in the NIMH Epidemiological Catchment Area Study. *American Journal of Psychiatry*, 148, 1494–1500.

Simon, G.E., Vonkorff, M., Piccinelli, M., Fullerton, C., & Ormel, J. (1999). An international study of the relation between somatic symptoms and depression. *New England Journal of Medicine*, 341, 1329–1335.

Singh, A. N. (2006). Role of yoga therapies in psychosomatic disorders. *International Congress Series*, 1287, 91–96.

Taylor, R.R., Jason, L.A., Richman, J.A., Toress-Harding, S.R., King, C., & Song, S. (2003). Epidemiology. In L.A. Jason, P.A. Fennell, & R.R. Taylor (Eds.), *Handbook of chronic fatigue syndrome* (pp. 42–72). Wiley.

Tulkin, S. R., & Gordon, M. (1998, August 14–18). Clinical health psychology in kaiser's redesign of adult primary care [Conference presentation]. American Psychological Association National Convention, San Francisco, CA, United States.

Valins, S. (1967). Emotionality and information concerning internal reactions. *Journal of Personality and Social Psychology*, 6, 458–463.

Williams, P. G., Colder, C. R., Lane, J. D., McCaskill, C. C., Feinglos, M. N., & Surwit, R. S. (2002). Examination of the neuroticism symptom reporting relationship in individuals with type-2 diabetes. *Personality and Social Psychology Bulletin*, 28, 1015–1025.

Yanh, B. Z., Zhang, H., Ge, W., Weder, N., Douglas-Palumberi, H., Perepletchikova, F., Gelernter, J., & Kaufman, J. (2013). Child abuse and epigenetic mechanisms of disease risk. *American Journal of Preventive Medicine*, 44, 101–107.

1 Theoretical Origins

The traditional biomedical model aligns with allopathic medicine, meaning "contrary to disease" in Greek. This model focuses on reducing or relieving symptoms. Holistic medicine, rather, emphasizes health promotion (*health*care rather than *sick*care), and recognizes many healing methods. Holistic medicine does not utilize a one-size-fits-all approach or suggest a specific treatment is always right. Instead, the best treatment is determined by the uniqueness of each individual's condition, context, and the functional and emotional factors associated with their symptoms.

Spirituality and Health

Historically, the practice of medicine has often integrated aspects of spirituality and religion. One could even claim the Buddha was a great early cognitive-behavioral therapist for suggesting that suffering is relieved with the right understanding and right action (Miovic, 2018).

However, in scientific communities today, "consciousness" may be the term that most approaches "spirit." (Scott, 1997). Despite the reluctance to emphasize spiritual ideas in evidence-based medicine, spiritual health is a known contributor to both mental and physical wellness (Carmody et al., 2008). Spiritual health is generally defined as peace of mind, trust or faith in life, a sense of compassion for and connection with oneself and others, a sense of purpose or meaning in life, and a transcendent awareness of self (Hayes, 2019). Including spirituality within medical care today is most often seen in the treatment of addictions (e.g., 12-step self-help programs) and end-of-life care.

Yoga

Practices for integrating spirituality and healthcare tend to follow many of the same principles as yoga, and several of the 12-steps even mirror principles of different yoga systems: devotion and prayer (bhakti), knowledge and meditation (janana), and action and work (karma) (Miovic, 2018). Each style of yoga emphasizes different practices and points of concentration for raising consciousness.

DOI: 10.4324/9781003251293-2

Western culture has traditionally viewed yoga as either a spiritual philosophy or a form of physical exercise. Since the 1970s there has been growing exploration of using yoga for psychological development and self-actualization (Ghei, 1976). The traditional intention of yoga is the "modification of one's self-awareness and relationship to the world. Yoga is a complete system of therapy, which includes developing awareness and control of the physical body, emotions, mind, and interpersonal relations" (Rama et al., 1976, p. 1). The purpose of yoga is to progressively expand one's consciousness by gradually, intentionally, and systematically integrating contents of the mind (in and outside awareness), which also leads to an expansion of one's self-definition. Yoga therefore involves both an evolution and an integration of the self. This is how yoga views psychological growth and development (Rama et al., 1976).

Energy

The yoga conceptualization of energy ("prana") includes both physical and mental energy. This energy is understood to be involved in all aspects of experience. There have been various theories that have focused on certain types of energy, such as psychic, mental, sexual, or bio-energy, but each represent a limited view of the energy field. Yoga, however, is a unified approach to exploring and understanding all forms of energy within the individual and their environment (Rama et al., 1976).

The study of energy is difficult to standardize or verify through traditional scientific measurement or observation. Western psychology prioritizes verbal forms of study and communication, which limits the ability to study that which is purely experiential. Through the practice of yoga, individuals focus their attention inward to explore their internal space, including their mental and physical processes. This introspection allows for the uncovering of an "internal map" of experience and energetic patterns (Rama et al., 1976). These "inner spaces", which Western traditions have struggled to observe and study, become accessible for observation through meditation and introspection.

Altering inputs of either mental or physical energy can be used to adjust the total energy levels and direct energy to a particular point of awareness (Cunningham, 1981). For example, certain postures and breathing exercises can modify physical energy levels, while some mental exercises of concentration modify mental energy. Either change creates a shift in the total energy balance. Many practices of yoga are understood as altering energy levels in this way (Rama et al., 1976).

Yoga Theory of Mind

Jnana yoga provides the most comprehensive understanding of psychological processes, which is based on the Vedic tradition and the teachings within the Prasthanatrayi (the *Upanisahds, Brahma Sutras*, and *Bhagavad Gita*). In jnana yoga, there are three aspects of the mind, each with their own purpose and yet they also function together as a whole. The first is the "lower mind" (manas), which gathers sensory information and organizes it with motor responses. It cannot evaluate the data it collects, so its tendency is to doubt and responses are based on habit, instinct, or impulse. The lower mind also coordinates and plans actions that are decided upon and ordered by buddhi, or wisdom. Next is the sense of "I" or "I-ness" (ahankara), which translates sensory-motor information into personal experience (e.g., *my* thoughts, *my* feelings). This is one's subjective sense of identity and personal distinction from that which is outside the self. This takes time to develop, as children are not born with a sense of "I", but rather utilize their parents or caregivers for this function. Without a developed sense of "I", an individual is very adaptable and flexible to various situations, but they are also greatly influenced by their environment. In some theories of psychology, this may be termed "ego", but in yoga this concept extends beyond the notion of ego. It is not an organization of the self, but simply the boundary which distinguishes "I" from "not I". Lastly, is wisdom ("buddhi"), which is the evaluation aspect of the mind. This is where the mind makes decisions, and uses discrimination and judgment to determine which response to engage. If buddhi is weak or under-developed, responses will be overly influenced by emotion, impulse, and prior conditioning (Rama et al., 1976).

Another mental structure is the memory bank ("chitta"), which stores all past experiences. Chitta has been compared to a stream which holds the flow of mental activity. Some psychologists may think of chitta as the "unconscious", a container for all history and data typically stored outside awareness. The contents of chitta, however, can "bubble up" in the lower mind, like projections on a screen, especially when outside stimuli and interference is controlled. "When nothing current or 'live' is being broadcast, then 'replays' and old movies are seen" (Rama et al., 1976, p. 58). Outside the mind, are the five senses which filter through sensory stimuli and then send selected information to the lower mind. Data is sorted according to one's operating self- definition. Information that is consistent with one's sense of "I" tends to be accepted and passed on to the lower mind, while information that does not fit the current self-concept is rejected. This "selective inattention" helps protect the individual by dismissing content that would be uncomfortable, or even painful, for the individual to integrate into their consciousness. However, this material maintains a constant threat to the individual's rigid and limited sense of self and reality. Often outside their awareness, the individual will be fighting to keep this material hidden away. This form of experiential avoidance wastes energy and furthers the narrowing of their frame of reference, field of decision-making, and repertoire of responses (Rama et al., 1976).

East vs. West

The different cultural styles and symbols of the East and the West have led to divergent understandings of yoga. In Western cultures, the ancient texts of yoga are generally viewed as spiritual and artistic rather than scientific and medical (Rama et al., 1976). Carl Jung is credited with popularizing yoga psychology in the West. He was intrigued by the observation that Hindu thought traditionally starts globally and reduces to applications at the individual level, while Western traditions make observations at the individual level and then attempt to generalize (Jung, 1976). Jung used the term yoga as a general reference to Eastern philosophy and medicine, and was specifically interested in yoga as a tool for spiritual personality development. However, Jung was careful to emphasize the symbolism rather than a literal interpretation of yoga texts, and understood these symbols from the framework of his own psychodynamic theory (Coward, 1985).

Yoga postulates that many mental processes occur outside of awareness, not unlike Freud's idea of personal unconscious or Jung's collective unconscious. In Jungian psychology, "the self" is an archetype within the collective unconscious, which is motivated towards integration and wholeness. The self in yoga psychology represents a blissful state of transcendence. Jung proposed the notion of collective unconscious, but maintained that each individual's consciousness develops separately from others, although they share guiding symbols. Jung's idea of "collective", is therefore quite distinct from the "transpersonal" concept in yoga. Transpersonal refers to the expansion of consciousness and one's sense of "I" so that the boundaries defining "I" are loose and permeable. In yoga psychology, individuals operating from lower levels of consciousness (e.g. sensory-motor mind) may appear quite different, and have different motivations and desires guiding their actions. However, as the individuals move into higher levels of consciousness, they are found to be increasingly similar. At the highest level of consciousness, their experience is actually shared (Rama et al., 1976).

Yoga is a "growth oriented" approach, in contrast to the Western disease-oriented approach. Western psychology uses diagnostic labeling to identify and categorize pathology, and applies intervention when a problem is detected. A yoga tradition emphasizes prevention just as much as early intervention, and conceptualizes distress as being due to skill deficits and needs for training. Yoga psychology is more of an integration of these two therapeutic approaches that engages both intervention for pathology and daily habits training, as well as behavioral and introspective methods of self-study and observation (Rama et al., 1976).

The Eight-Fold Path of Yoga

Most modern systems of yoga are based on Patanjali's systematic description of how one detaches from the contents of one's mind and expands consciousness towards self-mastery. This has been termed ashtanga (eight-limbed) yoga, or sometimes called raja yoga. Some refer only to the last four paths as raja yoga, and the first four as hatha yoga (Rama et al., 1976).

The eight phases are not completed in a hierarchical manner, but rather are simultaneously coordinated. Phases one and two involve developing regulatory control over everyday functions related to the body (niyama) and mind (yamas), or behavior and attitudes that promote moral discipline and purity. Phase three is meditation postures and positioning (asanas), and phase four is breathing exercises and control of breath (pranayama). With these hatha yoga techniques one is liberated from physical and mental tensions which inhibit mastery of the body. The individual then develops self-mastery skills by using breathing exercises to regulate energy.

Phase five is sense withdrawal or deprivation (pratyahara), in which voluntary sensory control focuses the mind to allow for greater observation of one's internal world. This internal focus quiets the external world, and, in this stillness, the contents of chitta (e.g. memories, images, emotions) enter one's awareness and can be integrated. The last three phases are extensions of one another in the process of achieving higher levels of consciousness: concentration (dharana) or single-pointed focus of the mind; contemplation meditation (dhyana); and highest consciousness (samadhi) or "perfect absorption of thought in one object" to release one's consciousness from the binds of the physical world (Singh, 2006, p. 92).

In the treatment of psychosomatic conditions, yoga approaches are usually based on hatha, mantra, or raja systems and emphasize the postures, breath control exercises, contemplation, and developing higher consciousness. Following a path of yoga is meant to help an individual integrate their personality; calm and focus their mind through modifying attitudes, motivations, and habits that influence health; and identify and pursue their central values (Singh, 2006). The benefits of a yoga approach to treating psychosomatic conditions include reduced tension and improved posture; relaxation; mental, emotional, and respiratory stability; enhanced blood flow distribution; and improved regulation of physiological processes (e.g., temperature, blood pressure, heart rate, oxygen levels, respiration). Psychologically, yoga facilitates greater awareness and self-understanding, which improves psychological well-being and protects against symptoms of anxiety, depression, and traumatic stress (Singh, 2006). When practiced appropriately, there are essentially no harmful side effects of yoga, highlighting the unique acceptability and wide potential of this approach. Yoga-based treatments are centered on activating one's abilities for self-regulation, emphasizing that the tools needed for health and wellness are intrinsic and personal.

Humanistic Psychology

Living organisms are programmed for self-preservation. When there is injury or illness, the human body will naturally attempt to heal itself.

However, sometimes the body's efforts to heal exacerbate the problem, such as in the case of autoimmune disorders or when bones heal incorrectly. The human psyche and spirit also naturally seek healing, but can similarly get lost or increase damage to the self along the way. Humanistic therapies rely on this innate and powerful self-healing capacity to treat psychological conditions.

Humanistic psychology is based on several assumptions regarding human nature. Firstly, humanistic psychologists view individuals holistically, believing that people cannot be reduced or compartmentalized into various subparts. Second, humans are conscious beings with an awareness of oneself, others, and their environment; meaning they construe their own reality based on their perceptions (Tudor & Worrall, 2006). Third, humans have will and the power of choice, which makes them responsible for their actions and circumstances (Rogers, 1989). Fourth, humans are experiential, directive, intentional, and meaning-making. This means they create goals, plans, and understand how their actions can impact future events. People learn through experience and seek to apply meaning to their past and present experiences. This also implies that an individual cannot be understood without consideration of their environment (Tudor & Worrall, 2006). Humanistic therapists work collaboratively with patients and believe that the patient holds the necessary wisdom and inner resources to achieve health and happiness (Rogers, 1989). Further, humanistic therapies emphasize the personhood of the client, the personhood of the therapist, and the therapeutic relationship throughout treatment (Scholl et al., 2014).

Humanistic psychology developed alongside phenomenology and the study of consciousness and experience. This included increased interest in the experiences of the body and acknowledgment of the body as a tool for personal growth. The therapy model proposed in this book is a whole-person approach to behavioral health treatment that utilizes the natural healing reflex of both the mind and the body to reduce psychological distress and promote self-development. In his book on integrative brief therapy, Preston (1998) writes that therapy helps initiate and direct the process towards self-development, but that this process continues beyond treatment and throughout life. Therapeutic interventions can help individuals re-enter their natural tendency towards greater health and healing, but it is this innate self-guide, not therapy, that will drive their direction and carry them through the challenges of life.

Carl Rogers: Client-Centered Therapy

Carl Rogers conceptualized psychological dysfunction as arising from individuals' maladaptive efforts to actualize and a lack of consistency (i.e. *incongruence*) between their self-concept and their experience. Rogers developed client-centered psychotherapy, which aims to facilitate the client's insight and help them achieve *congruence*. Congruence means that the individual's experience of themselves in the world (e.g. external actions and events, how they are treated by others) is consistent with their internal self-beliefs and self-attitudes, and that they are living and experiencing the most authentic version of themselves.

The role of the client-centered therapist is to hold appropriate attitudes with consistent techniques, but to not overly rely on directive methods (Rogers, 1951). The therapist seeks to understand the client's private world, but does not become immersed in it. Rogers believed individuals need to feel valued and understood in order to be able to integrate their experiences into their self-concept, and thus create an evolving and enriched sense of self. The warmth of the therapeutic relationship provides safety, which allows the client to feel vulnerable and explore their emotions and patterns. As the client explores various aspects of the self, the therapist communicates acceptance and understanding to help the client "listen to themselves" (Rogers, 1951), and then eventually acknowledge and repair inconsistencies causing distress.

Edward Tory Higgins: Self-Discrepancy Theory

E. T. Higgins (1987) expanded upon Rogers's idea of congruence/ incongruence and developed self-discrepancy theory (SDT) to increase understanding of how incongruence in one's self-concept can lead to unique cognitive and emotional patterns. Higgins's self-discrepancy theory suggests anxiety is rooted in a discrepancy between aspects of the self. SDT describes three primary domains of the self: the actual-self, the ideal-self, and the ought-self. The actual-self is an individual's subjective experience of themselves or true self-concept. The ideal-self and ought-self serve as chronic goals or "self-guides" that motivate and direct behaviors, emotions, and cognitions. The ought-self consists of the traits and attributes that one feels a societal obligation or responsibility (e.g., they *ought*) to possess, while the ideal-self is composed of the traits and attributes one most aspires for (e.g. would *ideally* possess) (Higgins, 1987). These self-guides can be adaptive or maladaptive depending on their development and use by each individual. The two main types of self-discrepancies in theory and research are actual-ought discrepancies (differences between one's actual-self and one's ought-self) and actual-ideal discrepancies (differences between one's actual-self and one's ideal-self). These two types of discrepancies are highly correlated (r =.50–.79), but have empirically and conceptually distinct functions (Boldero & Francis, 2000; Higgins et al., 1985).

An actual-ought self-discrepancy is a discrepancy between the attributes an individual thinks they should have and the attributes they believe they actually possess. It exists in the presence of perceived negative outcomes and generally leads to agitation-related emotions such as anxiety, fear, apprehension, guilt, and resentful anger at others (Boldero & Francis,

2000; Higgins et al., 1985). Physically, an actual-ought discrepancy may be associated with menstrual cramps, diarrhea, migraine headaches, and muscle cramps (Higgins et al., 1992). Cognitive restructuring may be the most effective strategy to match one's actual-self to one's ought-self guide (Boldero & Francis, 2000).

An actual-ideal self-discrepancy is a discrepancy between the characteristics an individual would like to possess, and those they believe they actually have. It exists in the perceived absence of positive outcomes and leads to dejection-related emotions such as dissatisfaction, depression, sadness, disappointment, and frustration/anger at oneself (Boldero & Francis, 2000; Higgins et al., 1985). Actual-ideal discrepancies predict feelings of doing less than desired and chronically unfulfilled hopes (Higgins et al., 1992). This type of self-discrepancy is more likely to be associated with stomach problems like nausea/vomiting, indigestion, and stomach acid (Higgins et al., 1992). An actual-ideal discrepancy is also negatively associated with self-esteem (Higgins et al., 1985). Behavioral strategies to match one's actual-self to one's ideal self-guide may be most effective (Boldero & Francis, 2000).

The greater the magnitude of a self-discrepancy, the greater the associated emotional distress and the interpretation of ambiguous stimuli as support for the discrepancy (Strauman & Higgins, 1987). When confronted with aversive self-awareness (i.e., a strong self-discrepancy), individuals are motivated to reduce the discrepancy or escape this negative self-awareness. However, their problem-solving strategies may prove maladaptive. Efforts to restore balance or reduce awareness can include harmful and/or avoidant behaviors, such as drug use, excessive or restricted eating, and other attempts to control one's experience (i.e., experiential avoidance).

Acceptance and Commitment Therapy

Acceptance and Commitment Therapy (ACT) is a behavioral treatment approach associated with the "third wave" of cognitive-behavioral therapy, and has been conceptualized as a client-centered approach to behavioral therapy (Hayes et al., 2012). ACT is also a mindfulness-based therapy which has helped to popularize the incorporation of Eastern philosophy into psychotherapeutic practices. Fundamentally, ACT utilizes acceptance and mindfulness processes and values-driven behavior change processes to increase psychological flexibility. The Society of Clinical Psychology (APA, Div. 12) has compiled sufficient empirical support to list ACT as an evidence-based treatment for a variety of conditions; including chronic pain, mixed anxiety disorders, depression, psychosis, and obsessive-compulsive disorder (American Psychological Association, Division 12, 2021).

The experiential model of ACT stems from philosophical roots in pragmatism, functional contextualism, and relational frame theory (RFT; Hayes et al., 2001). One key assumption of ACT is that human pain and suffering is universal, and arises from normal psychological processes which serve important functions (Hayes et al., 2012). It is perfectly normal for people to have unpleasant and distressing thoughts, feelings, and sensations. It would actually be quite concerning if someone was not having any of these experiences! The truth is that the highly evolved language and problem-solving skills of the human mind are not helpful in every context. These processes can be excellent tools, but people need to know when and how to use them. For example, symbolic language allows people to engage in sophisticated problem-solving, communication, and imagination tasks. These skills enable individuals to create mental images that are experienced as real despite them having no basis in reality (Hayes, 2019). This makes it easy to lose contact with the true present moment, and get caught in tangles of emotional distress and efforts to minimize this distress.

Extensive studies on RFT have demonstrated that human language is not learned through association (i.e., classical conditioning) as once hypothesized, but through elaborate networks of relationships. The human mind automatically derives bidirectional relationships between objects, symbols, and events in such a way that it can create an association between anything and everything. Some of these relationships are helpful (e.g., hot object = do not touch), and others are quite unhelpful (e.g., me = unlovable). This language ability of the human brain is amazing. However, due to many relationships forming outside of awareness, the mind sometimes generates unwanted or unhelpful thoughts or feelings that cause distress. People may try to get rid of a thought or remove a trigger, but no relationships can be deleted from these vast networks. What people *can* do is keep adding connections! Adding helpful relational frames and habits to these networks reduces the salience or importance of maladaptive connections, and facilitates moving in values-based directions.

ACT views symptoms as signals from the mind and body that a person's actions are misaligned with their values. Similar to client-centered clinicians, ACT clinicians tend to de-emphasize diagnosis and instead focus on the patient's current functioning. ACT philosophy focuses on treating the whole person rather than their symptoms(s), views people as stuck rather than broken, and maintains that all individuals have the capacity to move in a desired direction towards healing. Further, ACT highlights the role of experiential avoidance and the literal use of language (mental rules for behavior) as primary causes of symptomatic distress. The goal of ACT depends on what is functionally adaptive for the client (i.e., "workability"), insofar as a particular behavior is consistent with the pursuit of their stated values. In contrast to cognitive-behavioral therapy (CBT), which seeks to alter the *content* of thoughts and emotions, ACT aims to alter the *context* or one's relationship to thoughts and emotions. As a behavioral therapy, the ultimate goal of ACT is to engage in more variable actions that are values-based (Hayes et al., 2012). ACT proposes that no behavior is random, but is learned and reinforced. This means people have the power to make commitments and change their contexts in order to alter behavioral outcomes.

ACT is based on the psychological flexibility model (affectionately referred to as the "Hexaflex"), which consists of six core processes responsible for psychological health (flexibility): contact with the present moment, self-as-context, acceptance, cognitive defusion, connection with values, and committed action. The opposite of each process contributes to pathology through psychological inflexibility: attention to the past/future or inflexible attention, self-as-content, experiential avoidance, cognitive fusion, lost or distorted values, and impulsive action or inaction. Steven Hayes (2019), originator of relational frame theory and co-creator of ACT, writes that issues of psychological inflexibility arise from motivational life energies ("yearnings") that have become misdirected, and result in a narrowing repertoire of behaviors and ways of living. These yearnings are: belonging (self-as-context), orientation (present moment), feeling (acceptance), coherence (defusion), self-directed meaning (values), and competence (committed action). When attempts to fulfill these yearnings are misdirected, an individual may be defensive, lie, or hide in order to experience themselves as "special" (self-as-story); ruminate or worry (loss of flexible attention to the present), view life as a problem to be solved and attempt to impose false order with rule-based contingencies (fusion), avoid negative experiences of pain or discomfort and seek to feel good (experiential avoidance), pursue their wants or define their goals by "shoulds" and feel an emptiness or lack of gratification (fused, avoidant, or absent values), or seek external achievement, but struggle with procrastination or overworking (inaction, impulsivity, or avoidant persistence) (Hayes, 2019).

The "siren songs" of suffering within the psychological flexibility model are experiential avoidance and cognitive fusion (Strosahl & Robinson, 2008). Cognitive fusion refers to the entanglement of the self in cognitive processes (i.e., the inability to distinguish self from thoughts and other mental events), such that mental content is viewed literally. This leads to an overreliance on verbal constructs (e.g., rules) to direct behavior. Cognitive fusion produces action that is unresponsive to environmental contingencies and persists despite lack of success or even harmful consequences. Experiential avoidance is an attempt to alter the form, frequency, or situational sensitivity of an internal experience (Hayes et al., 2012), and includes distraction, numbing (e.g., substance use), and behavioral avoidance in response to distressing cues. Both cognitive fusion and experiential avoidance are used in efforts to control life experiences. ACT postulates that these control "solutions" are truly what cause and maintain distress. Common ACT interventions use metaphors and experiential techniques to help clients make contact with the present moment, improve perspective-taking abilities, deliteralize their use of language, practice mindful acceptance, identify their values, and choose values-guided behaviors.

Yoga has been practiced therapeutically as an experiential form of ACT, emphasizing psychological flexibility skills through movement and connecting with the body. In mindful yoga-based acceptance and commitment therapy (MY-ACT), the "science of ACT" is combined with the "wisdom of yoga" to discontinue the unworkable strategies people use to control or eliminate pain (Gordon et al., 2019). The creators of MY-ACT explain,

> Patañjali and relational frame theory help us understand why people suffer; Tantric philosophy, through yoga, meditation, breathing, and chanting, teaches us to focus our attention on concentrating more fully with the life we are living now; and functional contextualism provides us the truth criterion of function to evaluate how we are living and interacting with our suffering in a specific moment or context.
>
> (Gordon et al., 2019, p. 13)

ACT and Pain

In the context of pain, language and evaluating skills can add to suffering. For most animals, the experience of pain is time-limited to the actual presence of painful stimuli. Once the cause of the pain is removed, distress quickly resolves. Due to symbolic language abilities, the human experience of pain is not so limited. People can imagine pain, remember past pain, and anticipate future pain such that it feels like the pain is happening right now. Experiences of pain cannot be situationally controlled when the human mind can bring pain into any moment, any time, and anywhere. Imagination and symbolic language imply unlimited potential for suffering. This can lead to extensive patterns of experiential avoidance, as people seek to avoid any and all possible objects or events that could be associated with experiences of pain. It is not so hard to imagine how quickly this could take over one's life. These patterns are further exacerbated by cultural "feel goodism" whereby many seek experiences of pleasure and avoid those of pain (Hayes et al., 2012). When pain becomes persistent and distressing, people are encouraged to be curious and open to learning about their pain. Pain can teach an individual about their emotions and values. A popular ACT saying is, "you hurt where you care, and you care where you hurt" (Hayes, 2019, p. 24). Pain shows where one assigns value, and where they feel misaligned with a core value.

ACT for pain targets improved coping and daily functioning with pain rather than pain elimination. Attempts to suppress pain or distressing somatic symptoms are largely counterproductive and associated with increased pain perception and slower pain recovery (Cioffi & Holloway, 1993). The goal of ACT is to reduce pain-related distress and increase quality of life (Samani et al., 2019). As experiences of pain cannot be removed, the only option is to add experiences that increase effective coping, pain management, and values-based action. ACT may or may not alter the physiologic experience of pain, but reduces pain perception and subjective distress by decreasing the importance of pain (Smallwood et al., 2016). ACT may even help prevent acute pain from becoming chronic pain (Dindo et al., 2018).

ACT interventions for chronic pain help individuals learn to "take pain along for the ride" (Hayes, 2019, p. 369), and are associated with increased acceptance, satisfaction with life, and physical functioning; as well as reduced pain intensity, depression, and anxiety (Cederberg et al., 2016). Pain acceptance is the most empirically-supported mechanism of change of ACT for chronic pain. Acceptance correlates with decreased pain intensity, physical and psychosocial disability, depression, and pain-related anxiety and avoidance (Vowles & McCracken, 2008). Values-based action also mediates the effects of ACT for chronic pain. Along with acceptance, values-based action is negatively associated with pain-related distress, pain-related anxiety, depression, depression-related interference with functioning, and physical psychosocial disability (McCracken & Vowles, 2008). One study reported that pain acceptance and values-based action combined accounted for more than 50 percent of the variance in improved depression, more than 60 percent of the variance in improvements in pain-related anxiety, close to 40 percent of the variance in improved psychosocial disability, and more than 20 percent of the variance in improved physical disability. Learning psychological flexibility skills also lead to improved coping with pain at three-month and three-year follow-ups (Vowles et al., 2011).

In a study of 150 adults with chronic pain, McCracken and colleagues (2013) found that patients benefited from adopting an observer perspective, and making contact with their thoughts and feelings from this detached, defused stance. The authors found that two processes combined, pain acceptance and decentering, accounted for an average of more than 20 percent of the variance in outcomes measures of disability and distress, compared to an average of 2.5 percent of the variance accounted for by pain intensity. Decentering is a technique commonly used in mindfulness-based treatments. It involves observing thoughts and feelings from a detached perspective, and has been conceptualized as a combination of the ACT processes cognitive defusion and self-as-context. Through decentering, thoughts and feelings are understood to be temporary and not inherently meaningful or true. Decentering has been positively associated with pain-related acceptance, general psychological acceptance, and socioemotional functioning in individuals with chronic pain (McCracken et al., 2014).

ACT additionally decreases pain catastrophizing (Samani et al., 2019), a primary focus of CBT for chronic pain, despite ACT not actually targeting pain catastrophizing thoughts. Acceptance may also mediate the effects of pain catastrophizing on depression, pain-related fear, and physical and psychosocial disability (Vowles et al., 2008). Acceptance of pain catastrophizing thoughts involves an awareness of these thoughts as part of the pain experience without "buying-into" these thoughts or allowing these thoughts to alter one's mental or behavioral action.

ACT teaches individuals to give up the struggle for control with pain, observe pain with a willingness to experience it, and defuse from negative thoughts and self-stories about pain. Through ACT, people spend less time and energy on pain-related mental activity and instead focus on what matters most.

ACT and Stress

ACT has additionally been widely studied and used for stress management in both clinical and nonclinical populations. The psychological flexibility skills promote adaptive responding to any life event, and help improve coping with stress as well as reduce stress reactivity. Psychological inflexibility, on the other hand, moderates how stress and poor social support impacts physical and mental health. For example, one study found that as daily stress increased, individuals with low psychological flexibility reported a 60 percent increase in depression symptoms while those with high psychological flexibility reported an increase in depression of less than 6 percent (Gloster et al., 2017). ACT has also been found to encourage posttraumatic growth in patients managing long-term or chronic disease (e.g. cancer, multiple sclerosis, cardiac disease, HIV/AIDS) (Graham et al., 2016). When individuals are more effectively managing their stress through psychological flexibility, they also tend to engage in healthier habits not directly taught (Bond & Bunce, 2000).

All of the flexibility skills help reduce stress and the negative impacts of stress on health and other life domains. Defusing from negative self-perceptions or conceptualized goals/expectations also helps limit the impacts of stress. Perspective-taking skills build compassion for one's self and others who may contribute to or be impacted by our stress. Presence skills center attention in the moment, so that one's awareness does not get pulled into worries about the past or the future. Identifying values increases focus on what is most important, and committed action allows people to take steps towards desired change (Hayes, 2019).

References

American Psychological Association, Division 12 (2021). Psychological treatments. https://div12.org/treatments/.

Boldero, J., & Francis, J. (2000). The relation between self-discrepancies and emotion: The moderating roles of self-guide importance, location relevance, and social self-domain centrality. *Journal of Personality and Social Psychology*, 78(1), 38–52.

Bond, F. W., & Bunce, D. (2000). Mediators of change in emotion-focused and problem-focused worksite stress management interventions. *Journal of Occupational Health Psychology*, 5, 156–163.

Carmody, J., Reed, G., Kristeller, J., & Merriam, P. (2008). Mindfulness, spirituality, and health-related symptoms. *Journal of Psychosomatic Research*, 64, 393–403.

Cederberg, J. T., Cernvall, M., Dahl, J., Von Essen, L., & Ljungman, G. (2016). Acceptance as a mediator for change in acceptance and commitment therapy for persons with chronic pain. *International Journal of Behavioral Medicine*, 23, 21–29.

Cioffi, D., & Holloway, J. (1993). Delayed costs of suppressed pain. *Journal of Personality and Social Psychology*, 64, 274–228.

Coward, H. G. (1985). Jung and kundalinī. *The Journal of Analytical Psychology*, 30 (4), 379–392.

Cunningham, O. (1981). The relationship of psychic healing and insight oriented treatment within an expressive framework. *Pratt Institute Creative Arts Therapy Review*, 2, 15–24.

Dindo, L., Zimmerman, M. B., Hadlandsmyth, K., St. Maries, B., Embree, J., Marchman, J., Tripp-Reimer, B., & Rakel, B. (2018). Acceptance and commitment therapy for prevention of chronic post-surgical pain and opioid use in at-risk veterans: A pilot randomized controlled study. *Journal of Pain*, 19, 1211–1221.

Ghei, S. N. (1976). Introduction. In S. Ajaya, *Yoga psychology: A practical guide to meditation*. The Himalayan International Institute of Yoga Science and Philosophy of the U.S.A.

Gloster, A. T., Meyer, A. H., & Lieb, R. (2017). Psychological flexibility as a malleable public health target: Evidence from a representative sample. *Journal of Contextual Behavioral Science*, 6, 166–171.

Gordon, T., Borushok, J., & Ferrell, S. (2019). *Mindful yoga-based acceptance & commitment therapy*. Context Press.

Graham, C. D., Gouick, J., Krahé, C., & Gillanders, D. (2016). A systematic review of the use of acceptance and commitment therapy (ACT) in chronic disease and long-term conditions. *Clinical Psychology Review*, 46, 46–58.

Hayes, S. C. (2019). *A liberated mind: How to pivot toward what matters*. Avery.

Hayes, S. C., Barnes-Holmes, D., & Roche, B. (2001). *Relational frame theory: A post-Skinnerian account of human language and cognition*. Plenum Press.

Hayes, S. C., Strosahl, K. D. & Wilson, K. G. (2012). *Acceptance and commitment therapy: The process and practice of mindful change* (2nd ed.). Guilford Press.

Higgins, E. T. (1987). Self-discrepancy: A theory relating self and affect. *Psychological Review*, 94, 319–340.

Higgins, E. T., Klein, R., & Strauman, T. (1985). Self-concept discrepancy theory: A psychological model for distinguishing among different aspects of depression and anxiety. *Social Cognition*, 3(1), 51–76.

Higgins, E. T., Vookles, J., & Tykocinski, O. (1992). Self and health: How "patterns" of self-beliefs predict types of emotional and physical problems. *Social Cognition*, 10 (1), 125–150.

Jung, C. G. (1976). Psychological commentary on kundalini yoga. *Spring*, 1–31.

McCracken, L. M., Barker, E., & Chilcot, J. (2014). Decentering, rumination, cognitive defusion, and psychological flexibility in people with chronic pain. *Journal of Behavioral Medicine*, 37, 1215–1225.

McCracken, L. M., Gutiérrez-Martínez, O., & Smyth, C. (2013). "Decentering" reflects psychological flexibility in people with chronic pain and correlates with their quality of functioning. *Health Psychology*, 32(7), 820–823.

McCracken, L.M., & Vowles, K.E. (2008). A prospective analysis of acceptance of pain and values-based action in patients with chronic pain. *Health Psychology*, 27, 215–220.

Miovic, M. (2018). Integral yoga psychology: Clinical correlations. *International Journal of Transpersonal Studies*, 37(1), 199–225.

Preston, J. (1998). *Integrative Brief Therapy: Cognitive, psychodynamic, humanistic, and neurobehavioral approaches* (Vol. 1). Impact Publishers.

Rama, S., Ballentine, R., & Ajaya, S. (1976). *Yoga and psychotherapy: The evolution of consciousness.* Himalayan Publishers.

Rogers, C. R. (1951). *Client-centered therapy: It's current practice, implications, and theory.* Houghton Mifflin.

Rogers, C. R. (1989). A client-centered/person-centered approach to therapy. In Kirschenbaum, H. & Land Henderson, V. (Eds.), *The Carl Rogers reader: Selections from the lifetime work of America's preeminent psychologist* (pp. 135–152). Houghton Mifflin Company.

Samani, M. G., Najafi, M., & Boogar, I. R. (2019). Comparing the effectiveness of acceptance and commitment therapy and physiotherapy on quality of life and pain catastrophizing in patients with chronic pain. *Journal of Shahrekord University of Medical Science,* 21(6), 271–275.

Scholl, M. B., Ray, D. C., & Brady-Amoon, P. (2014). Humanistic counseling process, outcomes, and research. *Journal of Humanistic Counseling,* 53, 218–239.

Scott, B. J. (1997). Inner spiritual voices or auditory hallucinations? *Journal of Religion & Health,* 36(1), 53.

Singh, A. N. (2006). Role of yoga therapies in psychosomatic disorders. *International Congress Series,* 1287, 91–96.

Smallwood, R. F., Potter, J. S., & Robin, D. A. (2016). Neurophysiological mechanisms in acceptance and commitment therapy in opioid-addicted patients with chronic pain. *Psychiatry Research Neuroimaging,* 250, 12–14.

Strauman, T. J. & Higgins, E. T. (1987). Automatic activation of self-discrepancies and emotional syndromes: When cognitive structures influence affect. *Journal of Personality and Social Psychology,* 53(6), 1004–1014.

Strosahl, K., & Robinson, P. J. (2008). *The mindfulness and acceptance workbook for depression: Using acceptance and commitment therapy to move through depression and create a life worth living.* New Harbinger.

Tudor, K., & Worrall, M. (2006). *Person-Centered therapy: A Clinical Philosophy.* Routledge.

Vowles, K. E., & McCracken, L. M. (2008). Acceptance and values-based action in chronic pain: A study of treatment effectiveness and process. *Journal of Consulting and Clinical Psychology,* 76, 397–407.

Vowles, K. E., McCracken, L. M., & Eccleston, C. (2008). Patient functioning and catastrophizing in chronic pain: The mediating effects of acceptance. *Health Psychology,* 27(Suppl.), S136–S143.

Vowels, K. E., McCracken, L. M., & O'Brien, J. Z. (2011). Acceptance and values-based action in chronic pain: A three-year follow-up analysis of treatment effectiveness and process. *Behaviour Research and Therapy,* 49, 748–755.

2 Chakra Theory

Origins of Chakra Theory

Although less common in Western cultures, energy medicine has been practiced across the globe and dates back to many of the earliest societies and healing practices. A shared assumption in most Indigenous and ancient models of health is that only part of the human experience is physical (e.g., muscular, skeletal, respiratory), and that much of one's functional experience is actually energetic: chemical, electrical, mechanical, and subtle (beyond material). There is no limit to energy potential, and the way human energy manifests is highly variable and unique to each individual. Further, energy can be balanced or unbalanced, with either state producing diverse experiences physically, psychologically, and spiritually (Cunningham, 1981).

In yoga philosophy, there are three sheaths of the body. The first sheath is the physical body, and intervention at this level includes yoga postures, bioenergetics, and biofeedback. The second is breath and energy, which connect the body and mind. Relaxing the body creates a stillness that allows one to focus on breath. Similarly, breath regulation allows the mind (third sheath) to enter one's focus. There are five sheaths in total that make up the levels of awareness encapsulating the human experience. At the fourth level are altered states of consciousness, and the fifth level is a state of bliss (Rama et al., 1976).

The body's energy system also has three parts: aura (energy field), chakras (energy centers), and meridians (energy pathways). Meridians compose the system targeted by acupuncture (Nelson, 1994). Chakras are energy centers that form unique points of connection for the sheaths of the body (physical, energy, mental) to interact, or where consciousness meets the body. Translating into "wheel" in Sanskrit, the chakras are vortices where energy is at the highest concentration in the body, and various nerves center into plexuses. In ascending order, the chakras are understood as levels of consciousness or awareness increasing in complexity and expansiveness. Chakras continuously transmit and receive energy and transform life force energy into material energy. In Hindu traditions, this

DOI: 10.4324/9781003251293-3

vital life force energy is called "prana." There is no direct English translation, but in Chinese it is "chi" (e.g., tai-*chi*), and in Japanese it is "qi" (e.g., Rei*ki* and ai*ki*do) (Saradananda, 2018).

Maps of chakra-like energy systems within the human body have been found on all populated continents from ancient to modern times, indicating a strikingly similar and shared understanding of the human body and spirit across cultures (Best, 2010). Additionally, the caduceus, the medical symbol widely used even in the West, appears much like traditional yoga illustrations of snake-like consciousness and energy moving through the chakra system along the spine (Rama et al., 1976).

First described in writing over 4,000 years ago in Hindu religious texts, the Vedas, the chakra system was utilized in the ancient Indian system of medicine. Chakras became an integral part of Tantric yoga practices (beginning in India around 500 A.D), which combined the chakra system with kundalini yoga and became popular around the 6–7th century A.D. Tantra (also called Tantrism) is a word derived from Sanskrit for "web", and refers to a spiritual practice that views the body as a means for enlightenment, rather than a barrier. Tantra therefore integrates the physical body as a necessary component of spirituality. Hatha yoga was derived from Tantra, and includes purification practices (*sadhana*), postures (*asana*), and breathing control techniques (*pranayama*). Tantric systems of yoga are differentiated from Patanjali's *Yoga Sutras* in that Patanjali's approach seeks to transcend the body's "impure" physical form and desires. In Tantra, one actually focuses on the body and its passion as a path to enlightenment and self-realization (Coward, 1985).

Different systems of yoga may concentrate on particular chakras over others. Bhakti yoga, for example, seeks to transform the emotions of the lower chakras into a pure love in the heart chakra. Jnana yoga, on the other hand, focuses on the philosophical aspects of the two highest chakras for the development of wisdom. Other yoga practices focus attention on a particular chakra for meditation, such as in raja yoga, in order to achieve mental development and self-control (Rama et al., 1976; Singh, 2006).

Perhaps the oldest known book on the chakras is *Sat-Cakra-Nirupana*, written in Sanskrit by a Bengali yogi called Purnananda around 1550–1560 A.D. Sir John Woodroffe (under the pseudonym Arthur Avalon) translated this work and *Paduka-Panchaka* (10th century A.D.) into English, and included his own commentary and interpretations in his published book *The Serpent Power* (Avalon, 1918). Woodroffe also referenced another 10th-century text, *Gorakshashatakam*, which offers instructions for how to meditate on the chakras. C. W. Leadbeater followed in 1927 with his book *The Chakras*, which was largely based on his personal meditations. In the decades to follow, authors from a variety of fields, religions, and backgrounds would publish works on chakras and various uses of the chakra system, including several best-sellers. Anodea Judith is a somatic therapist and yoga expert who has published numerous books on the chakra system, yoga, and therapeutic healing, including *Wheels of Life: A User's Guide to the Chakra System* (1987), and *Eastern Body, Western Mind: Psychology and the Chakra System as a Path to the Self* (1996). Caroline Myss, a medical intuitive, published *Anatomy of the Spirit* (1996), to specifically highlight the role of chakras in physical health and medical healing. While there are many insightful and useful self-help books on the chakras, there is no education standard or regulation regarding who can make claims and publish works about the chakra system. This contributes to an abundance of literature that has not been critically evaluated and of questionable validity. This is a common and unfortunate circumstance in many branches of alternative medicine, where additional research is greatly needed.

Chakras open and close and energy shifts throughout daily experiences. Yoga practices of breath control, postures, relaxation, and meditation create deliberate energy shifts through the chakras and raise consciousness. Healthy energy flow through the chakra system is mirrored by physical and psychological health. Blocked, weak, excessive, or poor energy distribution through the chakra system manifests in physical and psychological illness (Cunningham, 1981). Knowledge of a patient's chakra system energies, therefore, has the potential to inform healthcare providers about the psycho-emotional-spiritual content that may be involved in their symptom presentation.

The Chakra System

The primary seven chakras are situated vertically up the spine and are associated with the endocrine and autonomic nervous systems (Best, 2010; Deekshitulu, 2014; Maxwell, 2009). Some yoga scholars write of additional core chakras and there may be more than 360 minor chakras (Best, 2010). However, these seven major chakras are generally believed to govern the entire system.

Chakras are described as physically connected by nadis, subtle threads of energetic matter. There are fourteen principal nadis, with three being the most important channels that weave through the entire chakra system: the ida, pingala, and sushumna (Avalon, 1918; Deekshitulu, 2014). In Western language, the sushumna has been linked to the central nervous system (CNS) with the autonomic nervous system running on either side. Life energy moves through chakras along the sushumna, similar to how the spinal cord relays electrical signals from the brain through the skeletal system. The parasympathetic nervous system has been associated with the ida and the sympathetic with the pingala (Deekshitulu, 2014). In most models, the chakras lie where these two nadis or pathways intersect and form plexuses (e.g., heart, diaphragm, and digestive system). Other models show the nadis crossing between the chakras instead of at them. It is important to recall that the chakras are subtle centers of energy and parallels between the chakra system and gross anatomy of the body should not be interpreted literally. Using physical and anatomical terms in the context of energy systems can be misleading. The chakras exist in the subtle (energetic) body, not the physical body (Goswami, 1999). When thinking of the body energetically, one almost has to learn a new language, with unique vocabulary and grammar rules (Rama et al., 1976). Some scholars have incorrectly stated that the sushumna, for example, is synonymous with the central spinal cord and that the ida and pingala refer to the parasympathetic and sympathetic nervous systems. The chakra and nervous systems are on separate energy planes and do not exactly map onto one another. However, using the language of the nervous system helps provide a symbol for Western cultures as to how the chakra system exists in the subtle body.

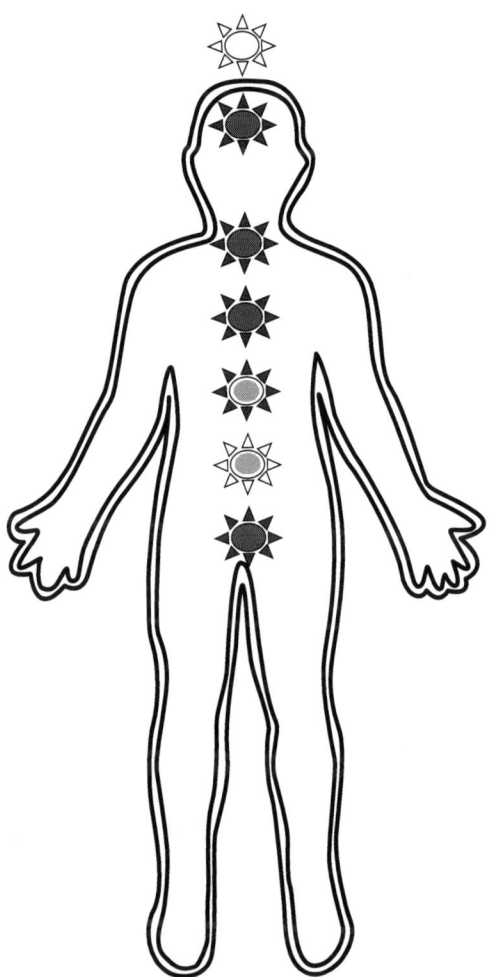

Figure 2.1 The Chakras

Modern Chakra Theory

In modern chakra theory, the chakras are interpreted as energy centers where life force integrates the mind, body, and spirit. The system functions as a hierarchy in that each chakra builds upon those below it, and the lower ones serve as a foundation for the entire system. This does not mean that those higher in the body are more or less important, but all are interrelated. The chakra system also corresponds with elements and colors. The elements for the seven primary chakras are earth, water, fire, air, sound, light, and thought. The colors are in the order of the rainbow: red, orange, yellow, green, blue, indigo, and violet or white (slower, longer vibrations towards faster, shorter vibrations). However, the original Tantric texts describe different color descriptions of the chakras as mostly various shades of red, yellow, smoky black, and white.

Anodea Judith (1987, 1996) describes two energy currents that move through the chakra system, one moving upward and the other downward. The upward current is the liberating current, and the focus of most chakra work. This energy is pulled by the spirit and mind, and flows from the root to the crown towards freedom, expansion, abstraction, and universality. This energy brings excitement and novelty, and is dynamic, expansive, and full of potential. The downward current she calls the manifesting current, which defines form, boundaries, and individuality. It has a systemic calming and organizing effect that brings a sense of peace and stability, and is pulled by the body and soul. The manifesting current produces grounding, which provides a sense of solidarity, safety, and connection. Physical pain, childhood traumas, sociocultural factors, and oppressive environments cut-off an individual from their grounding. Pleasure brings attention and awareness to the senses, and promotes expansion, while pain leads to constriction of the body and energy (Judith, 1987). A balance of both energy currents is needed. True enlightenment occurs after the individual has followed the liberating current upwards through the chakra, and then brings this enlightened consciousness back down through their energy system and applies it in their everyday life. Actualization of these two pathways brings connection, transformation, inspiration, and illumination (Judith, 1996).

Chakras and Physical Health

The chakras exist in the subtle body and also correspond with specific functions and regions of the physical body (Avalon, 1918). While highlighting the fact that the chakras are non-physical, Shyam Sundar Goswami discusses how the chakras influence "surface points" of the ventral body and "physical positions" of the chakras in the CNS (Goswami, 1999). Shrii Shrri Ánandamúrti (also known as Prabhat Rainjain Sarkar) refers to "concentration points" within the body associated with each chakra (Maxwell, 2009). Most relationships between the chakras and physical health are consistently reported, but there is some variation between scholars and yoga experts. This disparity is largely due to the interrelationships among the chakras, and the ability of a chakra to be stimulated through concentration points on parts of the body not necessarily linked with that chakra's location. This can create some confusion in the chakra literature as to where the chakras are located, where their concentration points are, and where else in the body the chakra may have influence (Maxwell, 2009). Further, the mechanisms by which chakras exert influence on the physical body is not well-specified, and is often described in terms of an "energy" or "force." Some of the autonomic nervous system effects of concentration on chakra points with yoga or meditation have been explained by chemical synaptic activity and the activation of the parasympathetic nervous system (Maxwell, 2009).

Generally, the physical aspect of each chakra is composed of three elements: a physical base in the dorsal CNS (along the spinal cord), a concentration point activating this physical base, and glands in the endocrine system which influence this physical base (Maxwell, 2009). Hormone secretions from endocrine glands alter mental and physiological functioning, and aim to maintain homeostasis or equilibrium/balance in the body. Like chakras, the different components of the endocrine system are functionally interconnected and influence one another. In order from root chakra to crown chakra, the chakras are typically associated with the adrenal glands, ovaries/testicles, pancreas, thymus, thalamus/hypothalamus, thyroid/parathyroid, pineal, and pituitary gland. Some scholars in chakra theory alternatively reverse the last two, and state that the brow chakra is associated with the pituitary gland while the crown chakras is associated with the pineal gland. See Table 2.1 for a summary of where each chakra exerts influence in the physical body. The seventh or crown chakra is not included as this chakra is purely spiritual energy.

Chakras and Psychological Health

Among the first scholars to Westernize the idea of chakras was psychiatrist and psychoanalyst Carl Jung, who viewed chakras as symbolic images in studying human consciousness and psyche (Jung, 1976). Jung presented a lecture series on Kundalini yoga at the Psychological Club in Zurich, Germany in 1932. He saw chakras as transcending time and the individual, helping to explain both the processes of an individual, but also the collective or universal consciousness of a culture or planet (Jung, 1976). Jung's understanding was that the chakra system could serve as a model for humans to develop higher consciousness. Jung expressed his belief that modern culture was stuck in a first chakra level of consciousness, a "prisoner in muladhara", where individuals struggle to see beyond

Table 2.1 Physical Aspects of the Chakras.

Chakra	Location	Endocrine System	Parts of the Body	Physical Dysfunctions	Sense
Root	Base of the Spine	Adrenal Glands	Lower spine (coccyx), feet, ankles, knees, rectum, bones, immune system	Chronic lower back pain, sciatica, varicose veins, autoimmune disorders (fibromyalgia, psoriasis, rheumatoid arthritis) leg/feet pain, constipation, osteoarthritis, obesity/weight problems	Smell
Sacral	Genital/ Pelvic Region	Ovaries/ Testes	Lower spine (sacrum), hips, sexual organs, large intestine, pelvis, appendix, bladder, prostate, spleen, kidneys	Obstetric/gynecological problems, pelvic pain, sexual impotence/infertility, cervical and uterine cancer, irritable bowel syndrome, urinary problems, lower back pain, lower gastrointestinal issues	Taste
Solar Plexus	Upper Abdomen	Pancreas	Middle spine, abdomen, stomach, small intestine, liver, gallbladder, pancreas	Gastric ulcers, colon/intestinal problems, pancreatitis, diabetes, pancreatitis, indigestion, anorexia or bulimia, liver dysfunction or hepatitis, metabolic problems, nausea, indigestion, gastritis, acid reflux	Sight
Heart	Center of Upper Chest	Thymus	Heart, chest, circulatory system, shoulder, arms, ribs, lungs, breasts, diaphragm	Congestive heart failure, myocardial infarctions, strokes, asthma/allergies, upper back/shoulder pain, shallow breathing or shortness of breath, bronchitis, high blood pressure, heart disease, breast or lung cancer, accelerated heart rate, hypertension	Touch
Throat	Base of Neck or Throat	Thyroid & Parathyroid	Throat, thyroid, trachea, neck vertebrae, respiratory system, mouth, teeth, gums, esophagus, hypothalamus	Raspy/sore throat, mouth ulcers, laryngitis, swollen glands in the neck, thyroid problems, chronic obstructive pulmonary disease, bronchitis, difficulty swallowing, feelings of choking, upper respiratory problems	Sound
Brow	Center of Forehead	Pineal	Brain, eyes, ears, nose	Brain tumors, migraines or headaches, sinusitis, neurological disturbances, stroke, blindness/deafness, full spinal problems, insomnia, seizures, glaucoma, vision problems, hearing or vision problems, tinnitus, myofascial pain syndrome, sleep disturbances, dizziness	All senses

their own impulses, instincts, and immediate physical experience (Coward, 1985; Jung, 1976). However, Jung used the framework of Kundalini yoga to communicate his own psychodynamic theory and ideas about the process of individuation, rather than to accurately describe yoga to a Western audience.

Chakra theory assumes that disease and dysfunction results from blockages within the system created by unresolved issues within the energy of a specific chakra. Blocked energy in one chakra can also force an adjacent chakra to overcompensate, resulting in an exaggeration of the neighboring chakra's positive energy and contributing to dysfunction (Nemri, 2004). Chakra blockages may occur as a result of trauma, injury, disease, mental or physical disorders, and situational factors that contribute to distress. Traditionally, different forms of yoga, breathing exercises, and meditations are suggested in order to resolve these energetic blocks (Avalon, 1918). Other common practices include vocalizations and sound work, mantras, journaling, and chakra drawing. See Table 2.2 for a summary of the central psychological themes of each chakra, psychological symptoms of distress, and therapeutic action that can restore healthy chakra energy.

Chakras and Developmental Stages

The chakra system has additionally been paralleled with human psychosocial development. Studying chakras in this context is meant to enhance understanding of both healthy and unhealthy developmental trajectories (Best, 2010). These patterns reflect either the flow or blockage of energy within a chakra and the greater system. In a chakra model of development, the goal-directed energy and activity of each chakra moves individuals forward to the next stage, as people are motivated to achieve equilibrium (Best, 2010). The chakra system represents an archetypal model of human maturation and goals and tasks associated with each chakra's energy reflect themes that are present throughout the human lifespan (Myss, 1996). Most developmental models of the chakras place the consciousness levels of the chakras on a lifespan continuum. Judith (1996) instead claims that individuals developmentally cycle through the entire chakra system by around age twenty with an external focus, and then cycle through again in adulthood with an internal focus and greater sophistication. Table 2.3 depicts a lifelong model of chakra development and includes parallels with Freud's psychosexual stages, Erikson's psychosocial stages, Maslow's hierarchy of needs, and Piaget's cognitive stages. The ages for Judith's (1996) model are italicized for comparison. The crown chakra is omitted because the crown chakra developmentally represents the experience of complete actualization. The chakras may parallel developmental stages, but are rather discrete domains of consciousness that individuals move through or transcend by embracing the lessons of each chakra's energy and integrating this growth into their experience (Best, 2010; Nelson, 1994).

Table 2.2 Psychological Aspects of the Chakras.

Chakra	Themes	Psychological Symptoms	Corrective/ Therapeutic Experience
Root	Survival Trust Family and Group Connection	Fear around primary needs, fear of loss, restlessness, anxiety, fatigue, hypervigilance, hypochondria, feelings of isolation/alienation, sleep or diet disturbances, chronic fatigue, low motivation, anhedonia	Establish safety/security and a sense of belonging; release attachments associated with fear; connect with physical and security needs; care for the body and the moment.
Sacral	Pleasure, Emotionality Control	Fear around secondary needs, social /separation anxiety, fear of losing control, obsessions & compulsions, indecisiveness, agoraphobia, restricted or excessive emotionality, limited/reduced pleasure in activities, guilt, self-blame/ blames others, restricted or excessive emotionality	Embrace change and let go of control; release attachments associated with guilt and blame; connect with flexible emotions and healthy pleasures; care for emotions.
Solar Plexus	Power Identity Responsibility	Fear of rejection/criticism, fears related to physical appearance or performance, nausea, low self-esteem, negative or disorganized self-concept, feelings of worthlessness, procrastination or avoidance of tasks, anger, shame	Assume self-responsibility; release attachments associated with shame and anger; connect with personal power/strength and self-esteem; care for convictions and attitudes.
Heart	Love Compassion Nurturance	Irritability, fear of emotional weakness/betrayal, jealousy, resentment, grief, avoidance or minimization of emotions, loneliness, tearfulness, restricted emotional experience/ affect, rationalizes emotions	Foster unconditional positive regard and empathy; release attachments associated with resentment and jealousy; connect with compassion (towards self and others); care for relationships.
Throat	Communication Creativity Choice	Anxiety regarding communication (e.g. selective mutism), fear of inauthenticity, hesitant, risk-avoidant, perfectionism, self-critical, tendency to focus on the negative, hopelessness, self-doubt	Embrace choice and creativity; release attachments associated with judgment, criticism, and doubt; connect with one's voice and truth; express oneself and listen to others; care for words and actions.

Chakra	Themes	Psychological Symptoms	Corrective/ Therapeutic Experience
Brow	Intuition Wisdom Imagination	Depressed mood, despair, attempts to rationalize depression or "think their way out," insomnia/hypersomnia, nightmares, inattention, poor concentration, ms, fixated on illusion of way things should be, sensory fears or hallucinations, derealization, depersonalization, fears of "going crazy"	Be open to new and alternative experiences; listen to one's intuition; release attachments of the mind (e.g. illusions, distortions, and fixations); connect with imagination; care for intentions and motivations (self-narratives).
Crown	Actualization Freedom	Fear of dying, existential anxiety or depression, overwhelmed by daily tasks, inner conflict about spiritual matters, feeling a lack of purpose or meaning, disillusioned with spirituality or extreme skepticism	Explore meaning-making; release all attachments; connect with universal consciousness; care for everything.

Chakras and Illness/Dysfunction

The chakra system creates a framework for understanding how different domains of energy interact and influence health. Each chakra has its own unique defining characteristics that differentiate its type of energy and power (Best, 2010). Good health comes from healthy chakras, but the system can become imbalanced or blocked for many different reasons, including stress, disease, traumas, and stagnant energy (Deekshitulu, 2014). The chakras therefore can offer a unique assessment tool for mapping symptoms and guiding treatment interventions to balance the mind, body, and spirit.

Many spiritual practices and ancient traditions propose that illness and distress come from depletions in one's energy and/or spirit. With this understanding, chakras can provide a sophisticated diagnostic system for almost any human distress or dysfunction (Nelson, 1994). Some yoga scholars suggest the challenges of each chakra be moved through in sequential order, embracing the positive attributes and energy of each before moving on to the next. This is partially due to the belief that without sufficient grounding in the first three chakras, the energy and lessons of the higher chakras could potentially become overwhelming or frightening, such as in manic or psychotic episodes (Nelson, 1994). Other yoga experts instead recommend targeting the higher chakras for developing higher levels of consciousness. Most often individuals will move between chakras in a varying order and at their own pace, even moving backwards through the chakras at times (Nelson, 1994). Whether each

Table 2.3. Chakras and Developmental Stages

Chakra	Ages (Judith's Model)	Freud	Erickson	Maslow	Piaget
Root	Infancy (0–24 months) *Womb-12 months*	Oral	Trust vs. Mistrust	Physiological	Sensorimotor
Sacral	Early Childhood (2–7 years) *6–24 months*	Anal & Phallic	Autonomy vs. Shame/ Doubt Initiative vs. Guilt	Safety	Preoperational
Solar Plexus	Middle Childhood & Adolescence (7–18 years) *18 months– 3 years*	Latency & Genital	Industry vs. Inferiority Identity vs. Role Confusion	Love and Belonging	Concrete Operational into Formal Operational
Heart	Early Adulthood (18–40 years) *3–7 years*	Genital	Intimacy vs. Isolation	Self-Esteem	Formal Operational
Throat	Middle Adulthood (40–60 years) *7–12 years*	Genital	Generativity vs. Stagnation	Self-Actualization	Formal Operational
Brow	Late Adulthood (60+ years) *Adolescence*	Genital	Ego Integrity vs. Despair	Transcendence	Formal Operational

chakra is active, underactive/blocked, overactive, or passively balanced determines how the chakra system will influence an individual's physical, psychological, and spiritual health.

Chakras are typically described as either opened or closed, and imbalance occurs when the energy of one or more chakras is excessive or deficient. An open chakra is able to receive and express energy, while a closed chakra is cut-off from energy flow. Chakra imbalances can be pervasive and/or persistent patterns in an individual's life or a temporary and specific response to a particular event. An excessively closed chakra is suggestive of a chronic avoidance, while an excessively open chakra may indicate a chronic fixation or overcompensation related to an unmet need (Judith, 1987; 1996). Both extremes on the continuum lead to problems with dysfunction and coping, as well as blocks in energy flow.

There are five primary categories of chakra blockages: physical, mental, intellectual, energetic, and karma (Saradananda, 2018). The first three types are most relevant to psychological treatment. Physical blocks indicate a need for basic self-care. The first step towards healthier chakras is working through the physical blocks by taking care of one's body with adequate sleep/rest, nutritious diet, regular exercise, and medical treatment for any physical ailments. Mental blocks are emotional, cognitive, and interpersonal patterns that interfere with an individual's actualization. Intellectual, mental, and emotional blocks can be conceptualized as aspects of psychological inflexibility, whereby rigid and maladaptive habits disrupt flow within the chakra system. Intellectual blocks occur when the analytic mind overpowers and an individual's thinking becomes literal and restricted. Energetic blocks are disruptions in energy flow through the nadi that prevent life energy ("prana") from reaching a particular part of the body, causing it to weaken and become sick. Lastly, karma blocks are related to the Hindu belief in past lives and that individuals may carry some of the energetic consequences of past actions.

Chakras and Incongruence/Self-Discrepancies

An individual's self-concept and understanding of the world around them matures and deepens as they learn to navigate the chakra system. The evolution of the self is the driving force pushing individuals through the hierarchy of chakra energy towards self-actualization, and integration of chakra energies allows for the formation of a complete and stable identity. In the language of humanistic psychology, the goal of yoga or chakra-based therapy is to achieve mind-body congruence, congruence within the self (self-integration), and congruence between one's values and actions. Distress, disease, and dysfunction are all manifestations of incongruence and maladaptive attempts to achieve congruence. Chakra blocks may also be conceptualized as types of self-discrepancies. As one energetically works with the chakras, they are confronted with many internal discrepancies (within the body, self, or actions) which forces them to either make a change that restores equilibrium or cope with the consequential distress. When people do not take action to repair the discrepancy, they become stuck in the associated chakra dysfunction, causing physical and psychological symptoms. The longer the imbalance remains in the body and the individual's psyche, the more likely it is to become internalized and understood as part of the person's identity. Further, what may start as a minor chakra imbalance can become a chronic, severe, or debilitating psycho-emotional problem and impact other chakras in the system.

Chakra Health and Healing

Broadly speaking, there are three methods of working with the chakras. The first is to physically engage with the chakras, including yoga, pos-turing and physical relaxation/stimulating practices. The second method is to focus on associated chakra features, which can be meditations on images, sounds, smells, elements, colors, etc. The third technique is to address the feelings and values connected with each chakra (Judith, 1987). Chakra-Organized Acceptance and Commitment Therapy (COACT) integrates components of all three methods, but particularly emphasizes the first and third to restore balance within the body, self-concept, and actions. Patients may explore other methods of working with the chakras, but clinicians should only practice methods within their competence. For example, it is common for people to work with the chakras through essential oils, crystals, or physical touch of particular points on the body. A behavioral health clinician should only incorporate those techniques in which they are appropriately trained and knowledgeable. COACT provides a practical framework for working with the chakras using empirically-supported behavioral health interventions. Each patient's chakra system must be considered as a whole, and chakras should be compared only to the other chakras in that same individual's system. It is only necessary that the individual be balanced within themselves, so comparing between individuals is uninformative and counterproductive.

The approach in this book is based on Acceptance and Commitment Therapy (ACT), and specifically targets increasing psychological flexibility in order to restore healthy chakra energy. ACT is not the only therapy that can be tailored to working with the chakras, but was selected because it shares many core ideas with yoga and Eastern philosophy. Further, the language of the psychological flexibility model aligns well with a conceptualization of dysfunction based on inflexible energy patterns and the idea that restoring flexibility and balance is key to improving health.

Research

During the 1970s and 1980s, interest in holistic and alternative treatments grew as individuals wanted to play a larger role in their health care (Harlan, 2001). In order to empirically explore these methods, the National Institute of Health (NIH) created the National Center for Complementary and Alternative Medicine (NCCAM) from the Office of Alternative Medicine in 1998 (Harlan, 2001). The language of complementary and alternative medicine (CAM) is often around dematerialization of the body (e.g., energy, chakras, auras, vital force, imbalances), in contrast to the biomedical approach which utilizes ever-evolving technologies to view, engineer, and control the physical body (Fadlon, 2004). Further, the majority of CAM approaches originated outside of Western culture. Healthcare providers today have commonly domesticated and modified CAM practices into hybrid treatments that are more familiar and acceptable to Westernized populations.

Many CAM treatments have empirical support; however, far more research is needed. Research and training of CAM that follows the biomedical model (e.g., shared terminology, laboratory demonstrations, scientific protocols to examine treatment effects) appears to help legitimize these practices for most modern healthcare professionals and many consumers (Fadlon, 2004). In a meta-analysis conducted by D'Silva and colleagues (2012), only 2 percent of the complementary and alternative medicine (CAM) studies found in a database search met their strict inclusion criteria based on the scientific rigor and quality of the study. The authors suggest that methods for evaluating medical treatments may need to be modified in the study of CAM approaches in order to accommodate their unique administration and change mechanisms. Maintaining the same quality of research and scientific rigor while studying treatments outside the traditional biomedical framework is an ongoing challenge for CAM researchers.

Due to these research challenges, there is limited scientific study of many emerging CAM approaches. However, a lack of scientific investigation cannot be used to make claims about the illegitimacy of any approach, as this says nothing about the model's empirical value (Jaenke, 2019). Nonphysical domains of consciousness and immaterial experiences cannot be scientifically proven or disproven by traditional methods (Miovic, 2018). Further, the field of psychology has always studied constructs and ideas that cannot be observed with the five senses. It is not necessary for us to "see" depression, self-esteem, or personality in order to work effectively with these ideas.

Chakra Research

While each chakra has distinct qualities, there is also overlap and cooperation between chakras such that no physical or psychological problem manifests from issues within only one chakra. The chakras are not mutually exclusive, which makes finding support for discriminant validity especially challenging and important. Knowing from which chakras a medical or psychological symptom originates could provide greater insight to the cause and how to heal the problem. For example, depression from the solar plexus chakra (lacking a sense of self and self-worth) would manifest differently than depression from the brow chakra (existential depression, hopelessness), yet they might share many common symptoms. Treatment that targets the unique properties of each syndrome would likely prove more effective than treating them the same.

The only published standardized measure of chakra energy is Caroline Myss's *Checklist of Health Issues and Illness* (CHII), a 74-item self-report instrument designed to inform subjects on the strength of their placements in each chakra (Myss et al., 2016; Schneider, 2004). The measure is largely a summary of the information in *Anatomy of the Spirit* (Myss, 1996) and Myss has not published reliability or validity studies on the CHII. In preparation for a dissertation study hoping to measure chakra energy qualitatively, Schneider (2004) conducted several analyses on the CHII and reported that the 74 items cross-correlated between domains and seven clear subscales did not emerge. Thus, while the CHII may be able to predict an individual's strongest chakra energy, it is not specific or empirically supported enough to be used as an aid in diagnosing the energy causes of varying disorders.

In her own attempt at measuring chakra energy, Schneider (2004) asked participants to respond to five essay-style questions and then coded their responses for analysis. Schneider (2004) called her measure the Assessment of the Chakras through Qualitative Responses (ACT-QR). The five essay prompts targeted different domains that were connected with specific chakra energies. As expected, Schneider (2004) found that most participants were dominant in the first three chakras, yet seven distinct subscales did emerge and support the discriminant validity of her questions and coding method. However, concurrent validity between the ACT-QR and the CHII was only found for chakra six (Schneider, 2004). Schneider also did not find expected correlations with well-established and widely-used measures to test concurrent validity of her chakra subscales, but concluded the measures selected were likely poor predictors of chakra energy and not variable enough to discriminate between chakras.

Clinical studies of the chakras to date have mostly been conducted by physicians and with the assistance of self-identified clairvoyants, medical intuitives, or others who claim the ability to observe the chakra system. Clairvoyant Dora van Gelder Kunz worked with nursing professor Dr. Dolores Krieger to develop the "therapeutic touch" technique that thousands of health providers have been trained in, and later co-authored a book with physician Dr. Shafica Karagulla, *The Chakras and the Human Energy Fields* (1989). In their research, van Gelder Kunz observed medical patients and described what she saw in their chakras, including the color, vibration, speed, brightness, shade, clarity, intensity, and size (Karagulla & van Gelder Kunz, 1989). Without previous knowledge of the patient's medical history, van Gelder Kunz reportedly observed energy changes and disruptions in the chakra system consistent with the patient's medical condition(s).

Other research has focused on working with the chakra system clinically to produce health benefits. A research team in Sweden provided an intensive course (14 hours a day for seven days) in mind-body and body-energy techniques to both men and women with baseline low health assessments, and examined health outcomes. The course taught how to achieve personal development through self-knowledge and supplemented it with information on the seven chakras. The course was found to have positive effects on health-related quality of life, including emotional well-being, cognitive functioning, sleep, and pain; as well as an increased sense of coherence (Fernros et al., 2008).

In Korea, 31 adults completed at least one of four weekly 30-minute meditation groups using *Caroline Myss' Chakra Meditation Music* (McNamara, 2002), and were compared to 32 adults who did not attend the meditation group. While all members of both groups maintained high levels of power and well-being throughout the study, those who attended the group were found to report increased power and well-being after two weeks of intervention. Those who did not attend actually reported a slight decrease in both power and well-being during the course of the study (Kim, Park, & Kim, 2008).

Health providers of diverse fields and backgrounds have additionally written about the potential benefits of a chakra-based model for such modalities as music/sound therapy (Balasubramanian et al., 2016), hydrotherapy (Nagaich, 2016), aromatherapy (Sreelakshmi & Manay, 2008), optometry (Berne, 2012), and dentistry (Sawicki, 2012).

Gilchrist and Mikulas (1993) developed a chakra-based model of group development in stages that parallel the developmental stages of Freud, Piaget, Eriksin, and Maslow. In this model, groups move through stages characterized by the prominent chakra themes: security, sensation, power, love, creativity/receptivity, integration/mindfulness, and fulfillment/ enlightenment. Gilcrhist and Mikulas proposed that during the security stage, group members need to establish a strong foundation and build rapport and comfort with one another. During the sensation stage, group members test boundaries, learn from their interpersonal interactions with one another, and engage in more emotional expression. During the power stage, group members work to resolve conflicts within the group and explore issues of self-understanding and control. During the love stage the group begins to feel cohesive as group members interact with mutual respect and compassion. During the creativity stage, the group is truly cooperating and engaging in shared creative problem-solving. Group members nurture one another and demonstrate openness and receptivity. During the integration stage, individuals engage in introspection to find their identity within the group. Finally, during the fulfillment stage, individuals experience a profound sense of unity with the group and both individual and group issues are resolved.

Lastly, this author's doctoral dissertation (Hale, 2019) developed a subjective self-report measure of chakra energy based on psychological themes associated with each chakra. The measure was titled the Chakra Energy Inventory (CEI), and consisted of seven chakra scales each with 13 items. The CEI chakra scales were found to have good internal reliability and construct validity. To examine the potential influence of the chakra system in disordered eating patterns, the CEI chakra scales were tested as predictors of anorexia-type and bulimia-type disordered eating behaviors in a nonclinical population. Self-discrepancies (actual-ought and actual-ideal) were further tested as possibly mediating the relationship between chakra energy and disordered eating behaviors. A composite variable of the lowest three chakras (root, sacral, and solar plexus) and actual-ought discrepancies both predicted anorexia-like dieting symptoms. Actual-ought discrepancies also partially mediated the relationship between these chakras and anorexia symptomatology. Additionally, actual-ideal discrepancies and a composite variable of the solar plexus, heart, and throat chakras both predicted bulimia-like symptoms. Actual-ideal discrepancies partially mediated the relationship between these chakras and bulimia symptomatology. These two mediation models support the role of poor chakra energy in the development of disordered eating patterns, and suggest that part of the chakra's influence is through self-discrepancies. The solar plexus chakra, associated with the gut and digestive system, was additionally found to be a unique predictor of disordered eating behaviors. This relationship highlights the role of such themes as self-concept, ego-identity, self-esteem, and personal power in the development of disordered eating.

References

Ánandamúrti, S. S. (1968). "This world and the next." In *Subhásita Samgraha*, Vol. 4. Ánanda Márga.

Avalon, A. (1918). *The Serpent power*. The Lost Library.

Balasubramanian, S. V., Balasubramanian, G., & Ramanathan, G. (2016). Integrative medicine system based on music. *Alternative Therapies in Health & Medicine*, 22, 14–23.

Berne, S. (2012). The science of measuring wellness. *Journal of Behavioral Optometry*, 23(3), 63–67.

Best, K. C. (2010). A chakra system model of lifespan development. *International Journal of Transpersonal Studies*, 29(2), 11–27.

Coward, H. G. (1985). Jung and kundalinī. *The Journal of Analytical Psychology*, 30 (4), 379–392.

Cunningham, O. (1981). The relationship of psychic healing and insight oriented treatment within an expressive framework. *Pratt Institute Creative Arts Therapy Review*, 2, 15–24.

Deekshitulu, B. (2014). Healing of chakras meditation on psychological stress. *Indian Journal of Positive Psychology*, 5(4), 398–402.

D'Silva, S., Poscablo, C., Habousha, R., Kogan, M., & Kligler, B. (2012). Mind-body medicine therapies for a range of depression severity: A systematic review. *Psychosomatics*, 53, 407–423.

Fadlon, J. (2004). Meridians, chakras and psycho-neuro-immunology: The dematerializing body and the domestication of alternative medicine. *Body & Society*, 10(4), 69–86.

Fernros, L., Furhoff, A.-K., & Wändell, P. E. (2008). Improving quality of life using compound mind-body therapies: Evaluation of a course intervention with body movement and breath therapy, guided imagery, chakra experiencing and mindfulness meditation. *Quality of Life Research: An International Journal of Quality of Life Aspects of Treatment, Care & Rehabilitation*, 17(3), 367–376.

Gilchrist, R., & Mikulas, W. L. (1993). A chakra-based model of group development. *Journal for Specialists in Group Work*, 18(3), 141–150.

Goswami, S. S. (1999). *Layayoga: The definitive guide to the chakras and kundalini*. Inner Traditions.

Hale, R. (2019). The influence of chakras on disordered eating patterns through body image self-discrepancies. [Unpublished doctoral dissertation]. University of Indianapolis.

Harlan, W. R. (2001). Research on complementary and alternative medicine using randomized controlled trials. *The Journal of Alternative and Complementary Medicine*, 7(1), 45–45.

Jaenke, K. A. (2019). Spiritual intelligence and the body. *ReVision*, 32/33(4/1), 71–82.

Jung, C. G. (1976). Psychological commentary on kundalini yoga. *Spring*, 1–31.

Judith, A. (1987). *Wheels of life: A user's guide to the chakra system*. Llewellyn Worldwide.

Judith, A. (1996). *Eastern body, western mind: Psychology and the chakra system as a path to the self*. Celestial Arts.

Karagulla, S., & van Gelder Kunz, D. (1989). *The chakras and the human energy field*. Theosophical Publishing House.

Kim, T. S., Park, J. S. & Kim. M. A. (2008). The relation of meditation to power and well-being. *Nursing Science Quarterly*, 21(1), 49–58.

Maxwell, R. (2009). The physiological foundation of yoga chakra expression. *Zygon*, 44(4), 807–824.

McNamara, S. (2002). Caroline Myss's chakra meditation music (Audio CD). Sounds True.

Miovic, M. (2018). Integral yoga psychology: Clinical correlations. *International Journal of Transpersonal Studies*, 37(1), 199–225.

Myss, C. (1996). *Anatomy of the Spirit*. Three Rivers Press.

Myss, C., Shealy, C. N., & Bruce, R. (2016). Checklist of Health Issues and Illness. Retrieved from https://www.myss.com/product/checklist-of-health-issues-and-illness/.

Nagaich, U. (2016). Hydrotherapy: Tool for preventing illness. *Journal of Advanced Pharmaceutical Technology & Research*, 7(3), 69.

Nelson, J. E. (1994). Madness or transcendence? Looking to the ancient East for a modern transpersonal diagnostic system. *ReVision*, 17(1), 14.

Nemri, K. (2004). Aiijii healing and how the chakras relate to disease and healing. *Proceedings (Academy of Religion & Physical Research)*, 36–42.

Rama, S., Ballentine, R., & Ajaya, S. (1976). *Yoga and psychotherapy: The evolution of consciousness*. Himalayan Publishers.

Saradananda, S. (2018). *Essential guide to chakras*. Watkins.

Sawicki, L. (2012). *Yin ain't yang: The ancient way to better health*. Lester Sawicki (Self-published).

Schneider, K. (2004). A qualitative and quantitative validation study of the assessment of the chakras through qualitative response (ACT-QR). California School of Professional Psychology, Fresno, CA.

Sreelakshmi, R., & Manay, N. S. (2008). Influence of aroma on human aura: Qualitative vibration of Pranas. *Psychological Studies*, 53(2), 137–145.

Singh, A. N. (2006). Role of yoga therapies in psychosomatic disorders. *International Congress Series*, 1287, 91–96.

3   Basic Principles of COACT

This chapter outlines an integration of yoga psychology and Acceptance and Commitment Therapy (ACT) to provide a summary of the basic principles of Chakra-Organized Acceptance and Commitment Therapy (COACT). Studies have found the psychological flexibility processes produce more specific and desired effects when contextualized to a particular concern or presenting problem (Carrasquillo & Zettle, 2014). COACT contextualizes the psychological flexibility skills of ACT within a yoga framework to treat psychosomatic symptoms. During COACT, the psychological flexibility skills are harnessed to heal the chakra system through somatic awareness, self-integration, and values-based action.

Spiritual Intelligence

Danah Zohar coined the term "spiritual intelligence" in 1997 and outlined twelve underlying principles: self-awareness (knowledge of one's values), spontaneity (attention to the moment), being vision-and value-led, holism (seeing the "big picture" and experiencing a sense of belonging), compassion, celebration of diversity, field independence (holding one's own convictions even if against the majority), humility, tendency to ask fundamental questions, ability to reframe (taking a step back and seeing larger context), positive use of adversity (learning/growing from pain and mistakes), and sense of vocation (feeling called to give or serve) (Zohar, 1997). Other definitions have emerged over the years, including David King's (2008) conceptualization of spiritual intelligence as a collection of mental capacities that facilitate the awareness, integration, and application of nonmaterial components of one's experience (Jaenke, 2019). King suggests there are four core components to spiritual intelligence: critical existential thinking, personal meaning production, transcendental awareness, and conscious state expansion. These principles of spiritual intelligence are strikingly similar to the principles of yoga psychology (Rama et al., 1976) and psychological flexibility (Hayes et al., 2012). Further, the chakra system can be used as a tool for developing spiritual intelligence through the body (Zohar & Marshall, 2000), and therefore may also be used to develop psychological flexibility. This is the foundation of COACT.

DOI: 10.4324/9781003251293-4

Mind-Body Relationship

Research has established that the mind-body relationship is bidirectional (Peper & Lin, 2012). In order to engage the healing abilities of both the mind and body, one needs to understand the inner workings of each, and how they interact. COACT aims to provide this framework in order to engage the mind-body connection and the self-directing ability of each to enhance health and healing, both physical and psychological.

In the United States and many Westernized cultures, individuals operate primarily from the mind and view the body as a tool; something the mind uses to accomplish goals and not in itself an important vessel for storing and retrieving information. Alternatively, the mind is rarely thought of as an instrument for the body to operate (Rama et al., 1976). Yoga helps individuals gain distance from both the mind and body in order to realize that the true Self is neither, and that both can be used for information processing and goal-oriented action. With this perspective, one can observe, regulate, and adaptively use their thoughts, rather than be controlled by them. Similarly, one can disentangle themselves from physical sensations in order to observe their functions (Jaenke, 2019; Rama et al., 1976).

Introducing a mind-body treatment approach to some patients may require early therapeutic work to help them feel safe and open to experiencing their bodies in a new way. There may be a learning curve and/or discomfort as a patient learns to build body awareness and make changes to the thoughts, feelings, and actions that contribute to physiologic sensations and symptoms (Bakal, 1999). It will be common for many patients to have managed their symptoms thus far on the basis of self-control and efforts to ignore their body. It may be counterintuitive, confusing, and even terrifying for them to begin reconnecting with the body. Building a safe therapeutic relationship and space is therefore imperative and forms an essential foundation for any intervention.

Yoga

Yoga means "union" or "joining together" in Sanskrit. The practice of yoga is the union of mind, body, and breath through physical postures, breath exercises, meditation, and relaxation (Spence, 2021). Within healthcare, yoga-based treatments are typically secular and emphasize general principles and practices rather than a particular system of yoga (e.g., hatha). Yoga views the body as the physical sheath of the self (Taittiriya Upanishad, 2020, 2.1), yet many individuals only attend to their body during experiences of pain or discomfort. When they feel sick or hurt, they are suddenly aware of their body and eager to "fix it." People generally assume an external cause (e.g., virus, bacteria, injury due to an outside object), and therefore seek an external solution (e.g., medication, bandage) that likely resolves an issue on the surface of the body. Once the superficial pain is resolved, most return their attention to the external world (Rama et al., 1976). This lack of attention to the internal functions of the body contributes to the challenge of understanding and treating psychosomatic illness. Many modern cultures do not encourage individuals to develop an awareness of their body, which would allow for receiving internal feedback and hearing the body's signals for help. Instead, people tend to believe that the functions of the body are outside voluntary control and unimpacted by choice and will (Rama et al., 1976). As long as these functions remain outside one's awareness, there is little one can do to change them.

The mental aspects of yoga include meditation, concentration, and self-observation. The only way to regulate the mind is to study the mental field through introspection, increasing awareness of each aspect and integrating it within the whole (Rama et al., 1976). Introspection requires separating the self from the contents of the mind, sometimes called the "observing self" or the "transpersonal self. It is impossible to observe one's inner activity while enmeshed with it. The goal is to look *at,* rather than look *from* the perspective of one's immediate mental experience. Observing from the mind tends to generate problem-solving, analyzing, and interpreting. This is what the mind does, and it does it well. However, this activity interferes with being present in the moment and the ability to witness one's experience unfolding. During the practice of introspection, "listening" refers to focusing attention and awareness to particular content in order to learn from it; "going into" refers to entering an experience consciously and voluntarily in order to allow the full expression of that feeling, thought, or sensation; and "understanding" refers to the ongoing balance of observing, listening, and going into processes (Miovic, 2018).

Kriya yoga is a beginner's style of yoga meant to prepare oneself for meditation and the practice of other, more advanced, systems of yoga. Kriya yoga involves engaging in self-study, austerity, and letting go of attachments to develop a higher consciousness (Ajaya, 1976). The practice of self-study means learning to view oneself with greater distance and objectivity. In this process, one discovers the difference between wants and needs. With this awareness, individuals identify patterns of attachment and release those that are not based on true needs. Further, as one expresses curiosity about internal events (e.g., thoughts, feelings, sensations, memories), they learn how this activity influences daily experiences. Through careful observation and detachment from experiences, an individual can identify with the true transcendent Self. Self-study leads to self-awareness, and then to self-realization (Ajaya, 1976). As one observes the thoughts and behaviors that contribute to discontent or energy imbalance, they have the opportunity and awareness to replace these habits with those that bring balance, joy, and contentment. In summary, the individual develops a stance of nonattachment in order to

1) enhance awareness; 2) connect with the transcendent Self; and, 3) choose actions that promote life satisfaction and healthy energetic flow. These represent the three key domains of COACT.

Nonattachment (Acceptance and Defusion)

Nonattachment reflects the capacity to observe one's self and environment with objectivity. To be unattached, is to "not get caught up and over-whelmed by the emotions, desires, or reactions of the moment" (Rama et al., 1976, p. 206). Nonattachment produces careful and curious observation of one's mental activity and environment which allows for greater choice in how one responds, as opposed to relying on automatic or emotionally-fueled habits. Practicing detached observation means one has to be willing to hold their awareness in the immediate moment and accept whatever is present. This means not trying to change, control, or alter their experience. Nonattachment is therefore a combination of cognitive defusion and acceptance.

Attachments, alternatively, are a blend of fusion and experiential avoidance. Attachments demonstrate where energy is caught or invested, such that it cannot move freely. Energy can be confined by rigid mental rules, expectations, or conceptualizations; as well as efforts to control one's experience to limit or eliminate pain. The terms "fixations" or "habits" are sometimes used synonymously with attachments. Attachments are fixed response patterns (behavioral, emotional, cognitive) upon which individuals build their self-understanding, and which guide their experiences. Attachments may be confused for values. However, attachments are inflexible and usually derived from social norms or cultural expectations (i.e., "pliance"), while values are flexible, freely chosen, and intrinsically meaningful to the individual (Hayes et al., 2012).

Letting Go

From the perspective of functional contextualism, the philosophical basis of ACT, truth is determined by function and how useful something is for achieving a particular goal. If something does not serve one's values or help them move in a desired direction, then it is not "true" or useful. Releasing these "false" attachments is the only way to make room for new possibilities. "If our hands are already filled, we cannot take on anything else" (Ajaya, 1976, p. 74). Further, one can let go of something mentally without needing to outwardly give it up. This means being able to enjoy an object or experience, while also knowing you do not *need* it. In other words, one's essence is not tied to that object or experience.

Contentment occurs in moments without any unfulfilled desires. When a desire shows up, individuals experience discontent or dissatisfaction until that desire is fulfilled. Discrepancies between one's current state and a desired state is what motivates action as they seek equilibration and a balance of desires. Many will spend their life pursuing an imaginary future where all desires are fulfilled and there is no more longing or discontent. However, basing one's life direction on external objects leads to patterns of seeking "good" experiences and avoiding "bad" or painful experiences. The biggest problem with this approach is that individuals will continuously chase after external objects and experiences meant to produce contentment, only to discover a new desire arises as soon as the last one is fulfilled. It is easy to get caught in a loop where the "finish line" (i.e., a state of total fulfillment) is a moving target, always just outside of reach. One may experience moments of satisfaction as they achieve each goal, but these moments quickly fall away as the next desire fills their consciousness. These attachment patterns lead to ongoing discontent and feelings of emptiness, while releasing attachments can help one give up this struggle and identify the source of contentment and peace within themselves (Ajaya, 1976).

Presence (Being in the Now)

The ability to stay present with one's experience is essential for being able to learn and grow from what is happening in the moment. Attention is like a flashlight for awareness; one's awareness follows where attention is focused (Hayes, 2019). The mind naturally pulls attention into the past or the future, seeking to evaluate, prepare, and make decisions. Feelings of insecurity or fear prompt individuals to get swept away by the mind's planning and organizing agenda. However, when one is entangled in worries and expectations, they are also removed from the joy and contentment available in the moment. Anxiety actually diminishes performance and effective action, serving as a barrier rather than assisting in the achievement of one's goals. A common adage states, "when you worry, you suffer twice." One can waste precious moments in anxious anticipation. Further, what could have been a positive experience becomes unpleasant due to anxious tension and worry about imagined scenarios. As an alternative to worrying, the best way to effectively prepare for any future situation is actually to center oneself in the now and take care of the present moment (Ajaya, 1976). Each response made in the present helps create the future.

Mindfulness

A widely used method for developing present moment attention is the practice of mindfulness. In yoga this might be called "meditation", but it is the practice of centering awareness on a fixed point in the present moment. The mind will naturally drift around and away from this point, and one can observe this process with curiosity and openness. It is important not to fight the mind's natural tendency, but to calmly notice the deviation and gently guide attention back to the point of focus (Rama et al., 1976). I often encourage my patients to imagine their mind is a puppy or small child that requires frequent, gentle redirection. Mindful presence is not losing oneself in the moment, but holding flexible, fluid, and voluntary attention to the moment (Hayes, 2019). If one experiences the moment fully, they become able to observe their patterns, build helpful habits, and continuously refocus their actions towards their values.

Mindfulness is also a practice of detachment and letting go, using defusion and acceptance skills to maintain present moment attention and counter experiential avoidance. As individuals become more aware of their habits and patterns (thoughts, feelings, behaviors), they have the opportunity to make intentional choices for their responses. Thus, mindfulness facilitates self-regulation of attention, while also encouraging individuals to reflectively respond to stressors and internal events. Mindfulness increases one's awareness of their internal processes, but the focus is on form rather than content. The individual observes these processes but tries to avoid interpretation or judgment.

Mindfulness-based treatments were not popularized and inducted as an empirically-based treatment in psychology until the early 1990s. However, Humanistic psychology's nonjudgmental acceptance combined with the rising interest in Buddhist themes in Western psychotherapy paved the way for mindfulness-based treatments to gain traction in research and clinical practice (Dryden & Still, 2006). There are various cultural approaches to mindfulness. In Buddhism, mindfulness is practiced to observe one's experiences and obtain enlightenment. Buddhists believe there is no self, as all things are one, so there is no distinction between the self and experience. An approach to mindfulness based on Tantra yoga focuses on observing the self as separate from one's experiences; to observe, accept, and detach from one's thoughts, feelings, sensations, and memories (Gordon et al., 2019).

Transcendent Identity (Self-as-Context)

There may be nothing more central to an individual's wellbeing as their sense of self or their identity (Rogers, 1961). Individuals experience various identities, which fluctuate with different roles and contexts, and possess a core Self that remains stable. This transcendent Self is the constant "I" that is not limited by self-conceptualizations or story-telling narratives (Hayes, 2019). Further, this self functions much like a light, illuminating the mind, body, and experiences (Ajaya, 1976). The true Self is flexible, fluid and an ever-evolving process. It is not stagnant or fixed content, but a changing manifestation of one's context, history, and present experience. It is also the product of multiple revisions, as different selves occur in different contexts, and all are possible in any single moment (Rosenbaum, 2021).

The transpersonal self is an element of the transcendent self. Personalities are unique and differentiate individuals from others. At the personality level there is a clear distinction between "I" and "you." At the transpersonal level, these boundaries are loosened to reveal that one is simultaneously "I", "you", and everything in between, as all is one (Green & Green, 1971). As consciousness expands further, beyond self-preservation and maintenance, into a transpersonal state, the individual is liberated from binds of fear and worry into a state of bliss and tranquillity (Rama et al., 1976). Yoga refers to this state as Samadhi, the highest level of consciousness where everything is seen from a true perspective of shared universal consciousness. "We see that the same inner light shines in all of us", similar to how many drops of the ocean reflect their shared source (Ajaya, 1976, p. 19). Each individual is understood to be a unique expression of the collective whole. This state does not result from lost self-awareness, but an expansion of both the self and awareness (Ajaya, 1976). Some people may feel a stigma or hesitancy to discuss their encounters with universal consciousness, yet these experiences of transpersonal awareness are common. Moments of awe or overwhelming emotion, such as observing a mountain or sunset, the birth of a child, or sharing in a collective and meaningful experience with others may produce such a sense of transcendent connection.

Green and Green (1971) define transpersonal psychology as the psychology of ultimate values. ACT shares this values-focus and seeks to promote greater connection with the transcendent self (self-as-context) through perspective-taking exercises. These interventions often consist of moving one's awareness across the three primary perspective-taking continuums: now/then, here/there, I/them. By experimenting with holding both ends of each continuum at once, individuals expand the boundaries of their self-concept (Hayes, 2019). COACT additionally emphasizes engaging the knowledge and wisdom of the body in self-development. Don Johnson, professor of transpersonal psychology and somatics at the California Institute of Integral Studies, describes three ways that somatic practices lead to transpersonal development: developing a flexible self-concept, developing the capacity for complete direct experience of the moment, and developing higher levels of awareness (Johnson, 2013). Each of these mechanisms reflects a component of awareness as conceptualized in the ACT framework, specifically the psychological flexibility skills of self-as-context and present moment attention (Hayes et al., 2012).

Expanding the Self

An infant has not yet developed boundaries for a sense of "I", and quickly and easily becomes fused with whatever is happening in the immediate moment. This allows infants to be readily adaptable, as they have no choice but to take cues from their environment in determining behavioral responses. Without any self-concept to serve as a reference point, each experience is all-consuming, and they experience both pleasure and pain in extremes. Yoga psychology suggests these early experiences form the basis of later attachment and aversion patterns, with much of life being oriented towards achieving and maintaining pleasure (Rama et al., 1976).

When an individual experiences pain or displeasure, they may feel a threat to their sense of reality or self, and engage in actions that seek to avoid or suppress this discomfort. The current self-definition is unable to reconcile their present pain with the acting self-story. In yoga terms, the inability of the current "I" or self-concept to hold the reality of their experience is described as a "failure of the 'I'" (Rama et al., 1976, p. 126). The individual may feel helpless or a sense of loss and/or disappointment, but this "failure" is really an opening that allows for a redefinition of the "I" to correct some of its previous limitations. A more mature self-concept is developed with broader boundaries, and creates growth. As attachments are gradually and systematically let go, one's identity is able to expand and become more fluid (Rama et al., 1976). This makes room in one's self-definition to accommodate all of their experiences, not just the desirable or pleasurable parts. This same process is repeated many times over the course of one's life. Rejecting or ignoring part of the self or experience (e.g., avoidance) depletes chakra energy, as does fusion with a particular self-story.

The external personality is essentially a "bundle of habits" that have been selectively weighted, either consciously or unconsciously, based on how one chooses to invest their energy (Rama et al., 1976, p. 142). These combinations of attachments create one's identity. Given that the self-concept is formed through learned habits, it can also be changed by altering one's habits (Rama et al., 1976). To rephrase in basic behavioral terms, you are what you do.

Replacement of Habits (Values Identification and Committed Action)

Yoga promotes conscious and deliberate actions, rather than automatic responses. This "self-mastery" involves building routines based on actions that fulfill one's values and sense of purpose. When operating from survival mechanisms or automatic responses, learning and knowledge of alternative responses is extremely limited. Actions are done with minimal consciousness, and without flexibility. For some animals, there is no other way for them to interact with their environment. However, for most mammals, and humans especially, instinctual actions are primarily used in emergency situations. In most other contexts, behaviors are learned and alterable. Responses can be programmed and re-programmed towards greater flexibility. Humans have reasoning abilities that allow them to evaluate their responses and decide which habits help them fulfill their goals, and change or create new habits accordingly.

The quality of one's thoughts and actions, whether conscious or unconscious, reflect attachments and contribute to energy flow or disruption

(Cunningham, 1981). When attachments give way to psychological patterns that are rigid and listless, energy flow is hindered and people may find themselves "going through the motions" without fully experiencing life. To overcome this lackadaisical lifestyle, one has to develop daily habits that ground them in the present moment and their values. The choice to consistently pursue one's values in each moment requires motivation by immediate and self-reinforcing rewards. The pursuit of freely chosen values is inherently rewarding, not a means to an end. If one is attached to a particular outcome or external reward, motivation will decrease. Values-based actions are not a result, but a process, a *way* of engaging in one's life. If focused on the outcome, people may yearn for some future moment of success, and miss opportunities for success happening right now. It is not uncommon for people to say things like, "I'll feel so much better once I get this job" or "I'll be happy when I get married and settle down." These attitudes postpone experiences of joy and contentment until an uncertain future time, meanwhile there are experiences of happiness and peace being missed in the present (Hayes, 2019). Habits are also self-fulfilling, such that actions that narrow one's experience lead to other limiting actions (e.g. avoidance, rule-based action). In this way, one's experience becomes increasingly restricted or increasingly flexible based on which habits are developed.

Daily Exercise

Systems of tantra yoga teach not to withdraw from Earthly human experiences, but to engage even in the mundane of daily activities to develop and expand consciousness. Habits form a sort of "home base", an internal central position from which one experiences the world (Ajaya, 1976). Some people worry there is more (even too much) they need to cope with if they actively engage in their daily life. This may even be quantitatively true. However, qualitatively the process for responding is the same regardless of the number or intensity of stressors (Ajaya, 1976). The solution remains to practice self-observation and center on one's core Self and values. Every moment of the day is an opportunity to be authentic and pursue one's values. ACT seeks to promote daily action in the direction of one's values and greater psychological flexibility in order to incrementally build values-based habits.

Karma and Responsibility

In yoga, it is understood that one's choices and actions have consequences for which the individual holds responsibility. Individuals are responsible for how they respond to each moment and experience, and thus are responsible for their circumstances. Each future situation is created by one's current choices, thoughts, feelings, and actions (Rama et al., 1976). This can be both a frightening and empowering realization as people recognize their power to change their circumstances; yet there may be apprehension about change and stepping into the unknown. Part of being consciously aware of this power is to notice one's automatic responses and ways they may limit their sense of choice or responsibility. This includes developing the ability to change one's perspective, assume a different role, and/or alter the script of interactions with others in ways that disrupt automatic patterns and replace them with conscious ones. Assuming this self-responsibility also requires recognizing the lessons in each experience.

Equanimity

The principle of equanimity is the choice to view all situations as an opportunity for learning and growing. People place themselves in situations that offer important and needed lessons that facilitate personal development. This includes painful events and experiences, which often serve as the greatest catalysts for growth (Rama et al., 1976). When individuals try to erase painful events or memories, they not only lose those learning opportunities, but they invalidate their own self and experience. Steven Hayes comments on his own experience, "I suddenly realized that by declaring to myself that my anxiety was invalid, I had, in effect, slapped my internal eight-year-old in the face and told him to *shut up* or *go away*" (Hayes, 2019, p. 103). This experiential avoidance is also a rejection of the self, and contributes to greater distress. Accepting the lessons in pain therefore also means accepting the self who is hurting. Both yoga and ACT conceptualize pain as a source of information, rather than a problem to be solved. Pain informs where self-care, gentleness, and kindness are needed; where values are placed; and where committed action can resolve experiential discrepancies.

Levels of Consciousness

A common aim of yoga practice is to achieve expanding levels of consciousness, and to experience everyday life from a perspective of higher consciousness. Yoga systems guide individuals to progressively integrate the levels of consciousness into a complete whole, so as to move beyond the distress which takes place at the lower levels. The process is simple, but requires focus and practice. The individual must unify the typically disparate parts of daily life into a cohesive experience, fully integrating the fragments of the self into a whole. Traditional forms of psychotherapy utilize a similar process of detaching from limited perspectives towards higher levels of consciousness (Rama et al., 1976).

The chakra centers are understood as different seats of consciousness within the body, each offering a unique perspective. If an individual experiences the world predominantly from the consciousness of one chakra, they will view their experience with primary reference to either basic survival/security, sensuality and pleasure, power, compassion, creativity, or intuition and understanding. It may be helpful for individuals to gain awareness as to which perspective is guiding them in most situations. Most of the time people are stuck in the lower needs and consciousness centers, such that anxiety regarding security, pleasure/pain, and power tend to govern most actions. When individuals are aware of this process, they can then choose to develop alternative styles of responding (Rama et al., 1976). A change in one's internal level of consciousness, however, does not always require a change in external behaviors. Ajaya quotes a Zen master as once saying, "Before I was enlightened, I chopped wood and carried water. Since I've become enlightened, I chop wood and carry water" (Ajaya, 1976, p. 101–102). It is not so much *what* we do that is key, but *how* and *why* we do it. This idea once again rings in functional contextualism. The function, rather than the content, of the action or experience is what determines its meaning and value.

Meditation

Meditation is the primary intervention of yoga psychology, and is a universal tool for health promotion, transcending across religions and cultures (Kim et al., 2008). Meditation operates similarly to most forms of psychotherapy in that conflicts and problems impacting the individual's life are carefully brought into awareness so that they can be unpacked, understood, and responded to. Empirical studies have found various forms of meditative practice to be effective in the treatment of medical and behavioral health conditions (Gotink et al., 2015). The physiological effects of meditation are generally the opposite of those found in the "fight-or-flight" response characteristic of anxiety and psychosomatic conditions.

Ajaya describes the process of meditation as "the practical study of how to deal with disturbing thoughts" (Ajaya, 1976, p. 40). Having intrusive or distressing thoughts during meditation does not mean someone is a "bad" meditator, but rather that these uncomfortable thoughts are entering one's awareness in order to be worked with. When disturbing or unwanted thoughts enter one's awareness, they actually become less powerful and influential over behavior. With awareness, the individual can observe the thought and make a conscious choice about how to respond in a way that supports their values (Ajaya, 1976). This process is essentially an act of defusion, whereby one's relationship with the thought is altered rather than the thought itself.

There is no single way to practice meditation, but the central components are focusing the mind on one-point of awareness (e.g., body sensation, feeling, word, image) and practicing nonattachment (Ajaya, 1976; Kim et al., 2008). Attachments foster separation from the true Self, and meditation helps to release these dependencies in order to reconnect with one's core Self and values (Ajaya, 1976). During mediation individuals suspend any judgment or evaluation of the thoughts or emotions that arise. Further, a single-point of concentration facilitates energy shifts within the chakra system, contributing to a greater level of awareness and consciousness (Cunningham, 1981). Meditation, often combined with breathing techniques, physical postures, and/or mantras, is used to clear energy blockages within the chakras (Jaenke, 2019).

Meditation in Action

The greatest value of meditation comes from how the practice is translated into daily activities of living. Someone may spend ten minutes each morning in quiet contemplation, but what about the rest of the day? Meditation can provide direction and purpose that helps individuals move through each day with an anchoring awareness of their true Self and values. Utilizing a mantra, prayer, or concentrating on breath can help stabilize this central reference. Imagine a wheel is spinning swiftly. If you try to focus on a single point of its outer rim, you are likely to become disoriented. However, you can easily maintain concentration on the center of the wheel (Ajaya, 1976). The practice of meditative action helps maintain a sense of internal stability as people encounter the unpredictable and ever-changing world around them. This inner stability allows for lessening attachments, and living more actively and effectively within one's environment (Ajaya, 1976).

Treatment Model

Chakra-Organized Acceptance and Commitment Therapy (COACT) seeks to engage individuals in a complete experience of their body, self, and life. Full satisfaction cannot be achieved through mental activity alone, but must be *experienced*. Enhancing this engagement is done through increasing psychological flexibility and detaching from rigid cognitive, emotional, and behavioral patterns. COACT fosters a general perspective of nonattachment, including an open and accepting stance towards one's self and experiences. COACT encourages individuals to learn how to "listen" to their body and inner self in order to facilitate self-development and meeting self-care needs through three primary processes: 1) somatic awareness; 2) self-integration (including contact with the transcendent self); and 3) values-based actions.

Treatment starts with developing an attitude of nonattachment through defusion and acceptance skills. Patients explore how rule-based and avoidant strategies have shaped and maintained their painful symptoms, as well as disconnected them from experiencing their body, self, and life. Three types of interventions target each of the primary processes: body-oriented, self-oriented, and action-oriented. These interventions are further contextualized to enhance the energy of specific chakras. Body-oriented interventions consist of mindfulness, yoga poses, breathing techniques, and other relaxation strategies that promote somatic awareness. These exercises are taught and rehearsed during clinic visits, as well as practiced at home by patients. Throughout treatment, the patient is encouraged to regularly check-in with their body and physical sensations. Self-focused interventions facilitate the patient in developing a self-concept that is flexible and whole, making contact with transcendent self, and increasing self and emotional acceptance. These interventions engage perspective-taking skills to help the patient expand their sense of self to make room for all of their experience, including pain. Through action-oriented interventions, patients learn to modify their behaviors in order to support self-development, life satisfaction, and values-congruent living. The patient is empowered to change mental and behavioral patterns that maintain their distress, and try something new to move towards living as their most authentic self. They practice engaging in activities that promote their health and wellbeing, and making choices more consistent with their values and goals.

Clinician Characteristics

ACT/COACT maintains many core principles of humanistic psychology, including a focus on the whole person, the unique subjective reality (i.e. context) of the individual, and an emphasis on the patient's innate capacity to self-heal. Clinicians communicate respect for the patient's autonomy throughout treatment and demonstrate Rogerian core therapeutic conditions of empathic understanding, unconditional positive regard for the patient, and genuineness. Further, clinicians seek to understand the context of the patient and their experience, as well as the meaning the patient has assigned to their symptom. The clinician should be careful not to make their own interpretation or assumptions about the meaning or underlying cause of the symptom (Bakal, 1999). Consideration of the patient's cultural perspective and symbols is essential. The clinician should never try to persuade or convince the patient of a particular point of view, but always come back to the basics of functional contextualism – what is true is what works for the individual in their context and moves them towards their values. It makes no difference what the clinicians think *should* work, or what *their* context and values would suggest, as this merely imposes rule-based contingencies and control efforts. The patient's life is their greatest teacher, and clinicians work within the framework of the patient's actual experiences (Strosahl et al., 2012). This experiential focus additionally means that treatment works with specific personal experiences rather than vague abstractions or generalizations (Freire et al., 2014). The patient is asked for detailed examples that help them to take a step back from their own experiences, and explore the thoughts/rules, emotions, and meaning they have attached to them. Through working with specific experiential accounts, the clinician and patient both achieve a better understanding of how the patient processes and responds to different events.

The therapeutic relationship is the most important tool in a clinician's repertoire. The primary function of the therapeutic relationship is to provide a context in which patients can learn new ways of interacting and being in the world according to their self-actualizing principles (Watson & Greenberg, 1998). In order for the patient to engage in these processes, they must feel safe and supported by the clinician. The clinician aims to foster a sense that they and the patient are working together and mutually involved and invested in the patient's therapeutic process (Freire et al., 2014). The therapeutic alliance should be egalitarian, non-hierarchical/horizontal, and collaborative. Patients and clinicians mutually agree upon goals and interventions of treatment, with each bringing in their own expertise. ACT highlights that a simple change in circumstances could reverse the patient-clinician roles ("there but for the grace of God, go I"), and clinicians hold humility and compassion for this reality (Strosahl et al., 2012).

A clinician further needs to be connected and grounded within their own body and experience in order to be fully present for the patient. If the clinician is avoiding or denying an aspect of their own self, they may find themselves uncomfortable or unable to effectively support the patient's process. The clinician may find themselves pulled out of the moment by their own thoughts, emotions, and physical sensations. Clinicians are humans too, and get caught by the same mental rules and pain-avoiding traps as anyone else. Clinicians are encouraged to practice psychological flexibility skills and meditation in their own life. The goal is not to be a perfect example of psychological flexibility, but rather to model acceptance, awareness, and turning towards one's values (Stroshal et al., 2012).

Patient Characteristics

COACT challenges a patient to take personal responsibility for how they have responded to their problems in the past, and make conscious choices for how to respond moving forward. This involves developing a strong and complete sense of self, as well as clearly defined values. During the initial evaluation, the clinician assesses the patient's readiness for COACT which includes the patient's level of psychological flexibility or willingness to develop greater flexibility. Other important aspects are the patient's willingness to recognize the limitations or unworkability of their current strategies, openness to trying something new, willingness to hold their painful experiences, use of control-based strategies, capacity for insight, and perceived sense of agency. A patient who is extremely inflexible in their thinking and behaviors is not necessarily a poor candidate for this treatment, but may require initial interventions more specifically focused on developing creative hopelessness and willingness to experiment with new strategies. Motivational interviewing techniques may also be helpful in assessing and increasing the patient's readiness for change.

Trauma Informed Care

Aligned with a model of Trauma Informed Care (TIC), the emphasis of treatment is not on what is wrong with the patient, but rather on what happened to the patient. Clinicians aim to place the patient's symptoms and distress in the context of their stressful life experiences, providing validation and normalizing their response. The basic principles of trauma-informed care are: Safety, Trustworthiness and Transparency, Collaboration and Mutuality, Empowerment, and Voice and Choice. Healthcare providers seek to establish a care environment that promotes open and reliable communication, provides respectful and person-centered care, engages in shared decision-making, demonstrates empathy and builds upon the patient's strengths, and validates the patient's autonomy (Substance Abuse and Mental Health Services Administration, 2014). Drawing upon the functional contextualism foundation of ACT, clinicians help the patient understand both the context and functions of their symptoms. It is not the patient who is broken or stuck, but their current strategies. Clinicians further demonstrate compassion and conceptualize the patient's symptoms as learned coping mechanisms and attempts to make sense of or survive extremely stressful situations.

Reducing Medication Use

Lastly, COACT and other behavioral treatments for pain aim to reduce the reliance on medications. Medications come with inherent risks for side effects, drug dependence, addiction, and dangerous interactions with other drugs. The current opioid epidemic largely grew from the overuse and over-prescription of pain medications, particularly for chronic pain. Long-term use of pain medication can actually worsen a chronic pain condition through increased sensitivity of the central nervous system. Further these medications are often counterproductive to goals for enhanced functioning and autonomy. The cycle of mental rigidity, experiential avoidance, fear of being without medication, and underutilization of behavioral and self-management strategies generally contribute to decreased functioning and ongoing distress (Bakal, 1999).

Reliance on medications can also lead to diminished confidence in one's own ability to manage their symptoms. With the belief that functioning is only possible with medication, people lose trust in themselves and faith that their behaviors could make a difference for their health. They may feel neither responsible nor capable of doing anything to improve their pain. This is not to say that there is no room for medication treatment, but that patients and providers should be mindful of the beliefs regarding medication treatment. What is harmful is the belief that the individual needs the medication in order to get through the day, and that without the medication they would be completely lost and unable to cope (Bakal, 1999). Pain medications are not cures, and they do not fix the underlying pain condition. Proper use of pain medication involves understanding the medication as a tool, ideally a temporary one, to facilitate accessing one's own inner resources for healing, such as listening to the body, learning behavioral strategies for coping with pain, making room for painful emotions, and engaging in values-based actions.

References

Ajaya, S. (1976). *Yoga psychology: A practical guide to mediation*. The Himalayan International Institute of Yoga Science and Philosophy of the U.S.A.

Bakal, D. (1999). *Minding the body: Clinical uses of somatic awareness*. Guilford.

Carrasquillo, N., & Zettle, R. D. (2014). Comparing a brief self-as-context exercise to control-based and attention placebo protocols for coping with induced pain. *Psychological Research*, 64, 659–669.

Cunningham, O. (1981). The relationship of psychic healing and insight oriented treatment within an expressive framework. *Pratt Institute Creative Arts Therapy Review*, 2, 15–24.

Dryden, W., & Still, A. (2006). Historical aspects of mindfulness and self-acceptance in psychotherapy. *Journal of Rational-Emotive & Cognitive-Behavior Therapy*, 24(1), 3–28.

Freire, E., Elliot, R., & Westwell, G. (2014). Person-centered and experiential psychotherapy scale: Development and reliability of an adherence/competence measure for person-centered and experiential psychotherapies. *Counselling & Psychotherapy Research*, 14(3), 220–226. https://doi.org/10.1080/14733145.2013.808682.

Gordon, T., Borushok, J., & Ferrell, S. (2019). *Mindful yoga-based acceptance & commitment therapy*. Context Press.

Gotink, R. A., Chu, P, Busschbach, J. J., Benson, H., Fricchione, G. L., & Hunink, M. G. (2015). Standardised mindfulness-based interventions in healthcare: An overview of systematic reviews and meta-analyses of RCTs. *PLoS ONE*, 10(4), e0124344.

Green, E. E., & Green, A. M. (1971). On the meaning of transpersonal: Some metaphysical perspectives. *Journal of Transpersonal Psychology*, 3(1), 27–46.

Hayes, S. C. (2019). *A liberated mind: How to pivot toward what matters*. Avery.

Hayes, S. C., Strosahl, K. D. & Wilson, K. G. (2012). *Acceptance and commitment therapy: The process and practice of mindful change* (2nd ed.). Guilford.

Jaenke, K. A. (2019). Spiritual intelligence and the body. *ReVision*, 32/33 (4/1), 71–82.

Johnson, D. H. (2013). Transpersonal dimensions of Somatic Therapies. In Friedman, H. L. and Hartelius, G. (eds) *The Wiley-Blackwell handbook of transpersonal psychology*. Wiley-Blackwell.

Kim, T. S., Park, J. S., & Kim, M. A. (2008). The Relation of Meditation to Power and Well-Being. *Nursing Science Quarterly*, 21(1), 49–58.

King, D. (2008). Rethinking claims of spiritual intelligence: A definition, model & measure. (Unpublished Master's Thesis). Trent University, Peterborough, Ontario, Canada.

Miovic, M. (2018). Integral yoga psychology: Clinical correlations. *International Journal of Transpersonal Studies*, 37(1), 199–225.

Peper, E., & Lin, I. (2012). Increase or decrease depression: How body postures influence your energy level. *Biofeedback*, 40(3), 125–130.

Rama, S., Ballentine, R., & Ajaya, S. (1976). *Yoga and psychotherapy: The evolution of consciousness*. Himalayan Publishers.

Rogers, C. (1961). *On becoming a person: A therapist's view of psychotherapy*. Constable.

Rosenbaum, R. (2021, March 11–12). Single session therapy (SST) [Conference presentation]. Removing barriers to integrated behavioral health in primary care: Research, best practices & implementations science (Interprofessional Primary Care Institute), Online. https://sites.google.com/marianoandassociates.com/ipc-institute/upcoming-events/behavioral-health-clinicians/advanced-mar-2021.

Spence, J. (2021). *Trauma-informed yoga: A toolbox for therapists*. PESI Publishing & Media.

Strosahl, K., Robinson, P., & Gustavsson, T. (2012). *Brief interventions for radical change: Principles & practice of focused acceptance & commitment therapy*. New Harbinger.

Substance Abuse and Mental Health Services Administration. (2014). SAMHSA's Concept of Trauma and Guidance for a Trauma-Informed Approach. *HHS Publication No. (SMA)* 14–4884. Rockville, MD: Substance Abuse and Mental Health Services Administration.

Taittiriya Upanishad (2020). Taittiriya Upanishad. https://shlokam.org/taittiriya (original work dated around 6th century).

Watson, J. C. & Greenberg, L. S. (1998). The therapeutic alliance in short-term humanistic and experiential therapies. In J. D. Safran & J. C. Muran (eds) *The therapeutic alliance in brief psychotherapy*. American Psychological Association.

Zohar, D. (1997). *Rewiring the corporate brain: Using the new science to rethink how we structure and lead organizations*. Berrett-Koehler Publishers.

Zohar, D. & Marshall, I. (2000). *SQ: Spiritual intelligence, the ultimate intelligence*. Bloomsbury.

4   The Chakra System

The Chakra System

Each chakra has a unique function and purpose, but they do not operate independently. Any chakra evaluation must consider the entire system. Similar to how a bodily system influences operations in multiple parts of the body (e.g. cardiovascular system), there is overlap and cooperation of chakra energy in determining physical and emotional functioning. Thus, while an anatomical structure or emotional experience might be primarily associated with a particular chakra, it is likely also influenced by other chakras in the system. Most problems arise from unresolved issues in the lower three chakras, because this is where most human energy lies.

Descriptions of the chakras commonly rely on symbolism due to the challenge of putting the experience of chakras into verbal language. This can be confusing for some seeking to understand the chakra system, especially those unfamiliar with the symbols of Eastern culture (Rama et al., 1976). The descriptions presented here, therefore, will not include the detailed visualizations and symbolism recorded in ancient yoga texts. For the purpose of treating psychosomatic conditions, this chapter will describe the areas of the body and central psycho-emotional attachments associated with each chakra. Attachments consist of rigid self-conceptualizations, emotional entanglements, and inflexible or distorted values, all of which contribute to narrowed behavioral responses and restricted life space.

Root Chakra (Muladhara)

The primary psychological themes of the root chakra are survival, trust, and family/group connection. The root chakra energy manifests as human beings' most fundamental needs and balanced energy in this chakra is essential for physical and emotional health (Best, 2010). When the root chakra is well-integrated, individuals feel solid and grounded (Cunningham, 1981). When this energy is poorly dispersed, individuals may experience fear or paranoia, and a sense of being unsafe in the world (Rama et al., 1976). The first chakra is associated with the element of earth, the color red,

DOI: 10.4324/9781003251293-5

and the sense of smell (Nelson, 1994). Healing the root chakra involves establishing safety, trust, and a sense of belonging; releasing attachments associated with fear; connecting with physical and security needs; and taking care of one's body and the present moment.

Body

Also called the coccygeal chakra, the root chakra is located at the base of the spine or the perineum. It serves as the foundation for the entire chakra system, and its location corresponds with the coccyx and coccygeal spinal ganglion, with minor chakras in the knees and feet (Judith, 1987). Areas of the body associated with this chakra include the lower spine (coccyx and lower lumbar vertebrae), feet, ankles, knees, rectum, bones, and immune system. The root chakra is also associated with the adrenal glands, which produce adrenaline for the body's "fight-or-flight" response to stress, secrete hormones for metabolization, and balance the body's salt levels. Common physical dysfunctions associated with this chakra are chronic lower back pain, knee pain, ankle/feet pain, sciatica, fatigue, auto-immune conditions (e.g., rheumatoid arthritis, fibromyalgia, psoriasis), and obesity/weight concerns.

Self

The root chakra represents the physical and grounded self. This is the self that is in tune with the body and physical needs for health and wellness. A primary orientation towards safety and survival can con-tribute to a preoccupation with physical health and bodily sensations, as well as a tendency to interpret routine or slightly unusual sensations as threatening. Unstable energy in the root chakra can also reduce somatic awareness and one's ability to receive communications from the body. As traumas associated with the root chakra cause disconnection from the body, restoring this connection and engaging the physical self is one way to restore energy to this chakra. This includes bringing awareness to the body through meditative practices (e.g., mindfulness, diaphragmatic breathing, yoga), as well as physical exercise and activity. Grounding is also important for a healthy root chakra. Grounding is a dynamic experience of feeling supported and bringing one's attention, focus, and concentration into the present moment. Mindfulness, the process of immersing oneself in the here-and-now, is one way of achieving grounding. Other strategies include engaging with nature, exercise, and self-care (e.g., eating well, sleep).

The primary task of the root chakra is to develop trust, as well as an internal assurance of emotional and physical security. This means making room for experiences of fear, and the self that feels afraid. Root chakra attachments commonly manifest as anxiety, nightmares, phobias, feelings of insecurity, illness/health anxiety, and hypervigilance. Fears associated with the root chakra are often global and intense, and may be disproportionate to the cause due to one's survival instinct being triggered (Schneider, 2004). Concerns include fear of abandonment and loss of physical order brought by sudden change (Myss, 1996; Nemri, 2004; Schneider, 2004). Fear is often maintained by avoidance (negative reinforcement), and therefore must be brought into awareness for one to work through it. Fixation of energy in this chakra leads one to be hypersensitive to events that may be perceived as an attack, and they may be quick to engage in defensive or self-protective acts. Often one can defuse the intensity of fear by learning to acknowledge and approach, rather than avoid, their anxiety. When people make room for fear and allow for its expression, they dispel the "fear of fear." By being willing to hold their worry and distress, individuals can also learn from it.

Through integrating fear, one also integrates the self who is afraid. Denial or avoidance of this emotion is similarly a rejection of the self who experiences it. Recall a time in which you felt afraid. Now try to recall what others said to you at the time. What was helpful and made you feel comforted and safe? What was not helpful and made you feel shut down or dismissed? Most likely, you felt better when your fear was validated and a loved one offered to help you cope with your fear. Alternatively, you may have felt more distressed if your fear was trivialized and you were told to "get over it." When people avoid or reject fear, they are essentially saying to themselves, "Your fear does not matter to me." How comforting is that? It is not surprising then, that this avoidant approach actually tends to increase distress. Control requires contact, so one must make contact with their fear and the self experiencing fear in order to provide themselves with the comfort and care that is needed.

Values

Values of the root chakra include family, group belonging, health, nature, order, physical activity, safety, self-care, stability, and trust. Actions that move people flexibly in the direction of these values help enhance the energy of the root chakra. When actions are inflexible, attachments of the root chakra may show up in fixed habits regarding conformity, safety, cultural or familial traditions and beliefs, or fitness/health. Strong motivations to move either toward or away from a particular experience are both forms of attachment. For example, firmly adhering to the rules and customs of one's family of origin and being uncomfortable with any variation is an attachment. Rejecting the culture one was raised in and harboring this animosity also reflects an attachment. Similarly, one can be neglectful of their body and physical health or have an excessive focus on it, and both represent attachments on opposite ends of a spectrum. Nonattachment comes from holding a flexible stance in the middle, where emotions, self-stories, and beliefs about what others might think or expect do not determine one's actions. Instead, actions are flexible pursuits of one's freely chosen values.

Sacral Chakra (Svadhisthana)

Central themes of the sacral chakra are pleasure/sensuality, emotionality, and flexibility/control. Sometimes called the pleasure or sexual chakra, this chakra governs psychological issues regarding blame/guilt, money, sex, and ethics and honor in relationships (Myss, 1996; Nelson, 1994). The second chakra has a theme of duality, including polarities and opposites attracting to create movement (Judith, 1987). The sacral chakra is associated with the color orange, the element water, and the sense of taste. Healing the energy of the sacral chakra involves embracing change and letting go of control; releasing attachments associated with guilt and blame; connecting with flexible emotions and healthy pleasures; and taking care of emotions.

Body

The sacral or spleen chakra resides in the genital/pelvic region below the umbilicus. Body parts associated with the sacral chakra include the reproductive system (e.g., genitals, ovaries, testicles, uterus), bladder, prostate, appendix, lower vertebrae, pelvis, kidneys, hips, large intestine, and spleen (Myss, 1996; Nemri, 2004). Common problems include chronic lower back pain (sacrum and lower lumbar vertebrae), genito-pelvic pain, hip pain, polycystic ovarian syndrome (PCOS), chronic pelvic pain, irritable bladder syndrome (interstitial cystitis), constipation, appendicitis, kidney or spleen dysfunction, and reproductive problems (e.g. infertility, impotence, pain with menstruation).

Self

The sacral chakra is associated with the emotional and playful self. Traumas associated with the sacral chakra cause disconnection from one's emotions. Emotional acceptance and connecting with healthy pleasures help restore energy in this chakra. A lack of engagement in enjoyable activities or fun will deplete this charka's energy, as will excessive pleasure-seeking. Individuals need to learn to embrace their feelings for all that they are, ambiguous and complicated, while also learning appropriate ways to manage emotions (Judith, 1996).

The emotional experiences of the self to integrate at the sacral chakra level are guilt and blame, as one learns how to explore desire and pleasure in healthy ways. Individuals are often taught by their culture to be wary of enjoying life's pleasures and encouraged to repress their experiences of pleasure in order to avoid overindulgence. They may believe that to be mature and responsible is to deny themselves pleasure and to feel guilty and remorseful about experiencing pleasure (Judith, 1996). This creates tension and pain physically and psychologically, which the experience of pleasure can release (Judith, 1987). Additionally, when healthy expressions of pleasure are denied, the body and mind may turn to harmful or dangerous sources of pleasure (e.g. drugs, excessive food, unsafe sexual practices, etc.).

Feelings of guilt and blame may be associated with issues of poorly expressed sexuality and self-gratification needs. An unsatisfying expression of sexuality is associated with physical dysfunctions (lower back pains, cramps, poor circulation, kidney problems), and emotional detachment (Judith, 1987). Issues with sexuality can include too much, not enough, addiction, shame, deprivation, compulsivity, and feeling unable or unsafe to express oneself sexually. Concerns about birth control, abortion, sexual orientation, relationship fidelity, celibacy, rape/sexual assault, and pornography, may be related to energy of the sacral chakra (Judith, 1996). Healing the energy of the sacral chakra involves balancing self-gratification and self-control, practicing moderation, and allowing oneself to seek pleasure and excitement in healthy and values-based ways.

Values

Values of the sacral chakra include adventure, beauty, control, excitement/fun, gratification, humor, pleasure, romance, sensuality, and sexuality. Actions towards these values require an openness to experience and willingness to feel. Otherwise, individuals may get caught up in trying to control or limit their experience by seeking only positive emotions or fun/happy memories. Sacral energy in particular motivates individuals to seek pleasure and avoid pain. This experiential avoidance not only removes the opportunity to learn from pain, but can also numb people to positive experiences. When one's emotional experience is limited, they lose contact with both ends of the spectrum, including joy, excitement, and passion.

Poor or disrupted sacral chakra energy is related to control efforts and attempts to regulate one's physical environment and relationships (Nemri, 2004). The "currencies of relationships" (Myss, 1996), sex, interpersonal power, and money, are most readily associated with the sacral chakra. Those with poor health in the sacral chakra may treat others as objects in their efforts to gain control over their environment.

Solar Plexus Chakra (Manipura)

The solar plexus chakra is the source of personal power and will. Central concerns of this chakra's energy include identity/self-concept, responsibility, and power (domination/submission). Building upon the matter/grounding of the root chakra and the movement (overcoming inertia) of the sacral chakra, the solar plexus chakra aims for transformation (Judith, 1987). This includes liberation from old patterns and creating new ones. The solar plexus is associated with the color yellow, the element fire, and the sense of sight. Healing of the solar plexus chakra involves assuming self-responsibility; releasing attachments associated with shame and anger; connecting with personal power/strength and self-esteem; and taking care of one's convictions and attitudes.

Body

The solar plexus or naval chakra is located in the upper abdomen and below the diaphragm. Problems within the third chakra can cause dysfunctions in the abdomen, stomach, small intestine, liver, gallbladder, pancreas, and middle spine; as well as issues of digestion and metabolism (Nemri, 2004). The endocrine system component of this chakra is the pancreas, which produces insulin and hormones to regulate blood sugar. Common health problems associated with the solar plexus chakra include abdominal pain, middle spine pain (higher lumbar and lower thoracic vertebrae), nausea, indigestion, gastritis, gastric ulcers, bloating, irritable bowel syndrome, acid reflux, dysfunctions of the liver (e.g. hepatitis) or pancreas (e.g. diabetes), and unhealthy eating habits (e.g. excessive eating, restricted eating, eating high sugar and/or high fat diets).

Self

The solar plexus chakra governs the powerful and responsible self. Traumas associated with the solar plexus chakra cause disconnection from one's sense of autonomy and an overreliance on the mind for guiding behavior. The latter refers to cognitive fusion, where thoughts are interpreted literally and individuals rigidly live by the rules or instructions of the mind even when their experience demonstrates these strategies to be ineffective or counterproductive. Connecting to the responsible self, entails taking accountability for one's actions and their consequences ("response-able" = capable of a response), and choosing responses that are more effective, efficient, and values-congruent. This choice is how individuals demonstrate their power. When people are disconnected from this aspect of the self, their actions may be dictated by automatic habits and rule-based contingencies, which contribute to feeling a lack of vitality, accomplishment, and purpose.

The strengths of the solar plexus chakra include self-esteem, self-discipline, ambition, strength of character, and the courage and ability to take risks and handle their consequences (Myss, 1996). All of these are hindered by the presence of shame. Shame and anger are the emotional experiences of the self to be integrated at the solar plexus level. Shame interferes with the ability to take personal accountability for one's actions and circumstances, while anger interferes with the ability to pursue one's goals responsibly and respectfully. Anger leads to impulsive and aggressive action, such that behavior is more emotionally-driven than values-driven. Both shame and anger are reactions to the belief that something "wrong" was done. With shame, this feeling is internalized such that the problem is believed to be within the self, while anger externalizes the problem. Both narrow one's behavioral responses, and limit perceived choices. Individuals may believe they "have to" act a certain way in order to be acceptable, or that they "must" retaliate in frustration to demonstrate strength. The solar plexus chakra has additionally been linked to Adler's concept of the inferiority complex, where one is distracted by concerns with adequacy, competition, and power (Rama et al., 1976)

Within the solar plexus chakra, there is an inner battle and struggle between the parts of the self that are approved of and the parts that are rejected or labeled "inferior" or shameful (Judith, 1996). This promotes fragmentation over integration of the self and depletes energy. Both shame and anger are determined by mental rules and beliefs about what "should be." People are ashamed of the aspects of themselves they do not want others to know or that they want to keep hidden, and feel angry when they perceive that someone has violated their rights or disrespected them. Anger is also a secondary emotion that commonly arises when a primary emotion is perceived as uncomfortable or unacceptable (e.g. fear, hurt, shame). These emotions may feel too vulnerable, so anger is used to feel stronger and more in control. People may experience anger towards someone who has hurt them, or called attention to their insecurities. They can also be angry with themselves for not behaving as one would like or failing to meet one's own expectations. Making room for experiences of shame and anger, therefore, involves releasing the rigid rules and attachments that limit one's self-definition.

Values

Values of the solar plexus chakra include assertiveness, challenge, courage, independence, persistence, power, responsibility, self-development, self-esteem, and skillfulness. Integration of third chakra energy helps to resolve problems with authority, aggression, pride, ambition, and competition (Cunningham, 1981). Balance of this energy also helps to establish self-confidence and self-assurance, which involves an honest recognition of one's strengths and weaknesses (Grubbs, 2016). An aspect of establishing individuality is developing autonomy and taking responsibility for one's self and actions. Solar plexus chakra energy is depleted when individuals avoid taking responsibility for their role in creating their circumstances (Myss, 1996; Schneider, 2004). It is also important for individuals to learn how to take effective and assertive actions to meet one's needs and goals while respecting the rights of oneself and others.

One's power is what allows people to act intentionally and actualize chosen potentials that help people create change and design their realities (Barrett, 1986). Power can be conceptualized similarly to Carl Rogers' idea of knowing participation, whereby awareness and freedom to act fosters knowing and intentional participation in the choices and changes people make as they interact with their environment (Barrett, 1986; Rogers, 1970). The goal is to use one's personal power from a place of unity and cooperation in order to protect and strengthen rather than control. Power without compassion (from the heart chakra) is a recipe for oppression, domination, and destruction (Judith, 1987). Attachments here may manifest as an authoritarian preoccupation with power, or someone who is passive, overly apologetic, and easily cowed. Alternatively, one could facilitate between these two extremes (Rama et al., 1976). Other attachments of the solar plexus chakra include body image/physical appearance concerns and competition/comparison.

Heart Chakra (Anahata)

The heart chakra is associated with love, nurturance, and compassion. Both the power and expression of love come from energy within the heart chakra, specifically unconditional love (Best, 2010). The heart chakra energy gives way to love for self and others, empathy, and forgiveness (Best, 2010; Cunningham, 1981). The heart chakra is associated with the color green, the element air, and the sense of touch (Nemri, 2004). Healing of the heart chakra involves fostering unconditional positive regard and empathy; releasing attachments associated with resentment and jealousy; connecting with compassion (towards self and others); and taking care of relationships.

Body

The heart chakra is located in the center of the upper chest behind the sternum. Dysfunctions within the heart chakra manifest physically in the heart, circulatory system, lungs, upper back (thoracic vertebrae), shoulders, arms, hands, ribs, chest/breasts, diaphragm, and thymus gland (Myss, 1996; Nemri, 2004). Diaphragmatic breathing helps balance the mind and body, and restores health in the heart chakra (Rama et al., 1976). The endocrine component of this chakra is the thymus, which is a lymphoid organ behind that breastbone that regulates T cells in the immune system. Examples of physical illness associated with the heart chakra include chest pain or heart problems, upper back or shoulder pain, arm pain, pain in the diaphragm or rib area, pain in breast area, shortness of breath or rapid breathing (i.e. hyperventilation), asthma/allergies, hypertension, accelerated heart rate, and postural orthostatic tachycardia syndrome (POTS).

Self

The heart chakra is linked with the compassionate and social self. This is the self that seeks deep emotional connections, and freely offers love, acceptance, and nurturance; the caregiving self. Traumas associated with the heart chakra are particularly likely to lead to disconnection from one's relationships and values. The heart chakra may be closed off due to trauma or other experiences of stress, protecting the heart from intimacy and connection. Making room for this part of self may feel vulnerable, as the openness of the heart chakra entails giving and sharing of oneself. However, with acceptance and self-compassion, individuals can hold this discomfort and move in the direction of their values. Practicing self-compassion involves nourishing the body, mind, and spirit through engaging in what matters. Values are intrinsically meaningful and require no justification or reason, much like selfless or unconditional love. People both love and value simply because they choose to.

Deficits in heart chakra energy can lead to barriers to forgiveness, such as jealousy, bitterness, and hatred. Grief is also an emotional experience of the heart chakra, and is an expression of love. People grieve for what is loved and lost, and grief is a reminder of one's love. These emotions interfere with the ability to demonstrate compassion, acceptance, and understanding towards oneself and others – they block one's heart. Individuals may focus their attention on others to deflect from a lack of self-acceptance, either pouring love into others when they cannot love themselves or needing a great deal of love and support from others. When these needs are not met, people feel defensive, alienated, and hostile. They may become consumed with their deficiency and experience self-centeredness to compensate for a felt lack of love (Judith, 1996). Healing the energy of the heart chakra allows one to build self-compassion and find this balance.

Experiences of jealousy and bitterness both reflect a sense of unfairness and scarcity. Scarcity refers to believing there is a limit to a desired object or experience. This means there is not enough for everyone, and that the more others have, the less there is available for oneself. If one is able to transition to a mindset of abundance, they can then release jealousy and resentment and replace it with compassion. Compassion also makes room for forgiveness. Forgiveness is not approving someone's actions, but recognizing their strengths and weaknesses, and allowing for who and what they are. This is a form of acceptance. When individuals can hold this stance of acceptance, they can bring compassion and move forward. They are released from the binds of bitterness, and get to choose where they want to put their energy instead; ideally, towards their values.

Values

The heart holds what is most treasured, and helps point individuals in the direction of that which they most value. Values of the heart chakra include compassion, empathy, equality, forgiveness, generosity, intimacy, kind-ness, love, relationships, and self-acceptance. The energy of the heart chakra focuses on one's internal world and emotional responses as it lifts one's consciousness above the more externally-oriented lower chakras. Love from the first three chakras is about filling a sense of emptiness, while love from the heart chakra comes from a sense of inner abundance and a genuine desire to share with others for mutual benefit (Nelson, 1994). Feelings of love and compassion within the fourth chakra are without the emotional binds of the lower chakras (e.g. viewing others as potential source of protection, threat, pleasure, or power), but there remains a distinction between self and other. Relationships tend to improve when others are appreciated for who they are and not what they can provide ("I need you" becomes "I love you") (Ajaya, 1976, p. 23).

Throat Chakra (Visuddha)

The throat chakra's energy is primarily related to communication (language and self-expression), choice, and creativity. This chakra is associated with a non-ego-based self and redirects some of the energy of the heart chakra in order to *receive* love, compassion, and grace (Best, 2010). The communication of the throat chakra includes artistic and symbolic expression. The throat chakra is associated with the color blue, the elements vibration and sound, and the sense of hearing (Nemri, 2004). Healing the throat chakra involves embracing choice and creativity; releasing attachments associated with judgment, criticism, and doubt; connecting with one's voice and truth; expressing oneself and listening to others; and taking care of one's words and actions.

Body

The throat or purification chakra is located at the base of the neck. Physical manifestations of problems in the fifth chakra appear in the throat, thyroid, trachea, neck vertebrae, mouth, teeth, esophagus, and upper respiratory system (Nemri, 2004). Examples of physical illness often related to the throat chakra include raspy/sore throat, mouth ulcers, neck pain, other mouth/throat pain, feelings of choking or difficulty swallowing, esophagitis, and chronic obstructive pulmonary disease (COPD). The endocrine components of the fifth chakra are the thyroid and parathyroid. The thyroid helps regulate metabolism and bone health, and the parathyroid regulates calcium and vitamin D.

Self

The throat chakra governs the honest and contributing self. This is the self that seeks to have a positive impact on the world and be a part of something meaningful. Traumas associated with the throat chakra cause disconnection from one's voice and integrity. Individuals may hold back and not express themselves fully, or they may express partial truths or fabrications. Expressing words that are not consistent with one's actions and values depletes the throat chakra. The throat chakra drives committed actions towards values, which requires integrity and an honest awareness of one's values. Individuals ask themselves not only *what* they want to do and be, but also *how* they want to pursue these goals (e.g., lovingly, passionately, dutifully, enthusiastically). This energy also guides moral principles and personal ethical codes. People develop a strong sense of self through the energies of the lower chakras, and the throat chakra helps them share who they are and what they have to offer with others and their environments.

The power of the fifth chakra lies in honesty and genuine self-expression; while dishonesty, insincerity, and self-criticism deplete the fifth chakra (Nemri, 2004; Schneider, 2004). The emotional experiences to be integrated at this level are doubt and judgment. With doubt, people experience a lack of conviction and certainty; while judgment stems from a false sense of certain authority. Both produce action that is lacking in integrity and honor. When people self-doubt or criticize, their responses are limited by beliefs about what they can or cannot do, rather than being guided by what they *want* to do according to their values. They put a limit on themselves and their choice of responses. Judgment similarly creates rigidly defined boundaries of acceptable behavior- both for oneself and others. These rules control and restrict one's own free and creative expression, as well as the ability to appreciate the unique expressions of others.

Resolving feelings of doubt and judgment involves compassionately releasing these attachments. Chastising oneself for experiencing self-doubt or holding a judgment is simply another manifestation of the criticizing pattern. These emotions are normal. The goal is to bring these experiences into awareness so that they do not unconsciously guide behavior. As an example, I am feeling a bit self-conscious about writing this book. I sometimes have thoughts of self-doubt, wondering if I am really knowledgeable enough to share this treatment approach, and judge myself for not writing more elo-quently. If I did not allow these emotions to enter my awareness, I may not be writing this book at all. My self-doubt and judgment could convince me to just give up, but then I would not be acting according to my values or pur-suing my passions with integrity. Tricky, isn't it? We need to integrate our feelings of doubt and judgment so that we can hold them, rather than them holding us.

Values

Values of the throat chakra include authenticity, community service, con-tribution, creativity, honesty, humility, industry, integrity, justice, and self-expression. This chakra is also associated with the idea of purity- purity of self and communication (Coward, 1985). Artists, musicians, and other creatives who use their craft to express their "true voice" are tradi-tionally believed to have high levels of energy in this chakra. It has further been suggested that the quality of someone's voice can be a partial indi-cator of their throat chakra energy. A voice that is constricted, whispered, or mumbled might suggest a weak throat chakra; while a loud, shrill, and interrupting voice may indicate an excessive throat chakra. A healthy throat chakra may correspond with a voice that is resonant, rhythmic, truthful, clear, concise, charismatic, and confident; as well as someone who listens as much as they talk (Judith, 1996).

The communication of the throat chakra includes not only what is expressed outwardly, but also the communication received and internalized from one's environment. This exchange is based upon the sources of information one puts their faith in (Rama et al., 1976). One's understanding of the world is largely derived from the media content (e.g. news, television, music, movies, websites) they are exposed to and seek out, as well as information internalized from social relationships and groups. Information without integrity weakens the fifth chakra, while media and content that enlightens helps heal this energy (Judith, 1987).

Brow Chakra (Ajna)

The brow chakra is associated with intuition, wisdom, and imagination. This chakra is also the center of cognitive functioning (Coward, 1985). When the mind is without clutter or confusion, there is opportunity for intuition and insight. Sensation and perception data is processed in the mind. When the brow chakra is healthy, perception is clearer and more reliable. The brow chakra helps individuals "see within" and observe their self and mind in order to notice anything which may be limiting their experience and shift perspectives flexibly and consciously. Individuals can also expand awareness to observe larger patterns or "the big picture." This pattern recognition requires the ability to simultaneously be attentive to the past, present, and future (Judith, 1996). The brow chakra is associated with the element light, the color indigo, and combines mental and spiritual energy for the sense of intuition (Nemri, 2004). Healing of the brow chakra involves being open to new and alternative experiences; listening to one's intuition; releasing attachments of the mind (e.g., illusions, distortions, and fixations); connecting with imagination; and taking care of one's intentions and motivations (self-narratives).

Body

The brow or third-eye chakra is located in the center of the forehead. Physical imbalances of the brow chakra manifest in the brain, sensory systems, sinuses, face, and head (Myss, 1996; Nemri, 2004). Examples include migraines, headaches, dizziness, insomnia, sensory dysfunctions, sinusitis, myofascial pain syndrome, and seizures (Schneider, 2004). The endocrine system component is the pineal gland, which produces melatonin and regulates the body's circadian rhythm and sleep cycle. It has been suggested that the brow chakra may function as the command center for the lower chakras, similar to how the pineal and pituitary glands influence other brain structures to control the endocrine system.

Self

The brow chakra governs the curious and reflective self. This is the self that seeks to know and understand. People gather information through their senses as well as through interoception (observing physiologic sensations) and introspection (observing mental processes). Traumas associated with the brow chakra lead to disconnection from one's intuition or inner wisdom. People may lose contact with or no longer trust their inner voice. They may even come to view the mind as their enemy, and seek to regulate and control the contents of their mind. Dysfunction in the brow chakra narrows perception and the ability to mentally step back from one's ongoing self-narrative. Connection with this aspect of the self brings the skill of flexible perspective-taking. This self is not limited by self-stories or conceptualized narratives, but rather plays with the ideas of truth and reality. What is "true" often depends on a number of contextual factors, such that what is true from one perspective may not be true from another. This self has the ability to consciously shift awareness into different times, places/situations, and people, to explore different possibilities. The self as this level of consciousness has expanded and holds loose boundaries of definition.

Emotional experiences in the brow chakra are deep and reflective. The emotional experiences to be integrated at this level are depression and despair. These emotions produce a dullness of the senses that can feel like a black cloud fogging up the mind, and limit the ability to see one's experience in multiple ways. Depression has many diverse symptoms, but includes a low mood and/or diminished interest or pleasure in life or activities. Joy and vitality are lost, and it can be difficult to see a path forward. Experiences of despair, which may accompany depression, involve a sense of hopelessness. Attachment to hopeless beliefs is dangerous, and a risk for suicide. These attachments narrow perception such that individuals become unable to imagine any alternative perspectives.

Making contact with these emotions may be painful and even frightening. People may worry about their ability to cope with these dark emotions in their awareness, and avoidance of these emotions is common. The ineffectiveness of labeling these emotions as "unacceptable" and trying to ignore or remove them will likely increase a sense of hopelessness, as this strategy is doomed to fail. Acknowledging and facing these emotions may help diffuse their intensity. I use the analogy of the boogey-man with my patients. When something only exists outside of awareness, it can be as terrifying as the limits of your imagination. However, once something is brought into awareness, its true form often feels less overwhelming. This awareness also allows one to start exploring and eventually letting go of the conceptualizations and self-stories that have imprisoned them. Further, it is important to hold compassion for the self that has been so confined as one experiments with new possibilities.

Values

Values of the brow chakra include awareness, clarity, curiosity, gratitude, imagination, knowledge, mindfulness, open-mindedness, spirituality, and wisdom. The challenge of the brow chakra is to open one's mind and detach from fused narratives in order to form an unbiased perspective from which to view oneself and the world (Myss, 1996; Nemri, 2004). The state of consciousness within the brow chakra opens a level of insight and intuition previously inaccessible (Best, 2010). This sort of detachment does not mean a lack of investment or uncaring, but a fearless and conscious presence inside the current moment. From this center of awareness, one can give up illusionary "false truths", connect with the voice of inner wisdom, and have the confidence to act on intuition (Myss, 1996). Actions that move people in the direction of brow chakra values include various forms of mindfulness, meditation, and spiritual practice that develop an internal focus of awareness. Sharing new experiences and learning about different topics also expand awareness and imagination. As one develops the ability to imagine alternatives, potentials, and hypotheticals, they shift from a narrow perspective to one with infinite possibilities. With this flexibility, knowledge gets transformed into wisdom (Judith, 1987).

The brow chakra is depleted by illusions and fixed narratives that distort or limit perception. Personal illusions are the stories that create self-fulfilling prophecies, and keep people confined to a particular path. Individuals may be attached to a particular narrative of themselves or others, and therefore all experiences are interpreted from this lens. People often believe these stories are fixed and predetermined. People may say, "That's just the way I am" or "It is what it is," as a means of deflecting personal responsibility. The idea of releasing a strongly held story may even be terrifying. One might think, "If I am not defined by this, then who am I?" Even when a story is hurtful, it provides something to cling on to. The idea that the self is variable, flexible, and contextual can be confusing and overwhelming without sufficient grounding. Grounding attention in the moment and developing the observing self-perspective helps center awareness for expanding the boundaries of self-definition.

Crown Chakra (Sahasrara)

The crown chakra is the highest state of consciousness and represents complete actualization and freedom (Best, 2010). At this level, there are no limits and awareness is expanded beyond description in verbal language (Rama et al., 1976). There is no I/you, here/there, now/then; instead, everything is one. Descriptions of this chakra are largely symbolic, as sahasrara is an experience, and one of complete connection or "cosmic consciousness" (Rama et al., 1976). This consciousness, once achieved, can be drawn back through the chakra system, enhancing integration and awareness at each chakra. The crown chakra is either violet or a glowing white (Nemri, 2004). Healing of the crown chakra involves exploration of meaning-making, releasing all attachments, and connecting with universal consciousness.

Body

The crown or unity chakra is located at the top or crown of the head where divine or life force energy enters the body and disperses throughout the chakra system. This spiritual energy does not typically manifest in physical symptoms, but has been associated with the cerebral cortex, nervous system, muscular system, skeletal system and the skin (Myss, 1996; Nemri, 2004). The endocrine component of the crown chakra is the pituitary gland, commonly referred to as the "master gland" for its regulation of several other glands and hormonal secretion.

Self

The crown chakra governs the transpersonal and universal self. This is the self that experiences connection with everyone and everything without boundaries. From this perspective, one deeply realizes that all is one. Traumas associated with the crown chakra cause a sense of disconnection from this universal source. This may result in a spiritual health crisis, rather than a physical or mental health condition. The crown chakra is the source of all consciousness, and allows for infinite awareness and enlightenment (Judith, 1987).

The emotional experiences of the self to be integrated at this level are existential angst and awe. As one explores and integrates all the physical, emotional, mental, social, authentic, and imaginative aspects of one's experience, the expansion of the self challenges them to question and release all attachments held at each level. As people let these attachments go, it is natural to wonder what is left? If the meaning of life and one's self-definition are not bound up in these attachments, then how does someone find purpose and meaning? Why are we even here? What even is here? What even is "I"? The sense of limitlessness that begins with flexible perspective-taking in the brow chakra becomes true limitlessness in the crown chakra. This can be an overwhelming experience, as one struggles to merge an awareness of the universal and infinite self with one's physical experience. Individuals may wrestle with their own mortality and fears about what does or does not happen after this life. These questions have always been part of the human experience. Integration of this angst does not mean any answers are found, but rather that one is willing to hold these questions even without answers. As the sense of universal connection is developed, one begins to feel more comfortable accepting that they may only have one piece of the puzzle, yet trust in the divine energy holding it all together.

Many feel a sense of universal connection during moments of awe. Experiences of awe occur when an individual lets go of all attachments in order to bring their awareness completely into the present. People might hold this sense of awe as they observe a sunset, view upon the mountains, participate in a meaningful social movement, witness life being born, or look into the eyes of a loved one. These are the moments in which one senses they are held and connected to some shared energy, spirit, or consciousness that is guiding their experience.

Values

Values of the crown chakra include freedom, spiritually, nonattachment, and self-actualization. In this chakra, one retains all of the knowledge and lessons of the previous chakras, and is totally free of all attachments, fears, and preoccupations; allowing them to unlock the highest human potential (Best, 2010). The ability to open oneself so fully to all of life's experiences demonstrates faith and psychological flexibility. Many believe only a few of the most enlightened and devoted spiritual leaders ever reach the stage of the crown chakra, while others believe this consciousness is too divinely governed and mystical for any human to reach in their lifetime (Nelson, 1994). Greater awareness and consciousness are gained through the crown chakra with meditation, devotion, and prayer (Myss, 1996; Nemri, 2004). Discouraging children (and adults) from such questioning and answer-seeking can deplete crown chakra energy, such as spiritual abuse, age-inappropriate structured religions, and religious practices forced on an individual (Judith, 1996).

ACT and the Chakra System

The psychological flexibility model of ACT includes six core processes. As a parallel, the crown chakra can be conceptualized as the larger domain of psychological flexibility, and the other six chakras each represent one of the core processes. The root and brow chakras promote awareness through present moment attention and flexible perspective taking (self-as-context). The sacral and solar plexus chakras foster openness with emotional acceptance and cognitive defusion. Lastly, the heart and throat chakras encourage engagement with values identification and committed action.

References

Ajaya, S. (1976). *Yoga psychology: A practical guide to mediation.* The Himalayan International Institute of Yoga Science and Philosophy of the U.S.A.

Barrett, E. A. M. (1986). Investigation of the principle of helicy: The relationship of human field motion and power. In V. M. Malinski (Ed.), *Explorations on Martha Rogers' science of unitary human beings* (pp. 173–184). Appleton-Century-Crofts.

Best, K. C. (2010). A chakra system model of lifespan development. *International Journal of Transpersonal Studies*, 29(2), 11–27.

Coward, H. G. (1985). Jung and kundalinī. *The Journal of Analytical Psychology*, 30 (4), 379–392.

Cunningham, O. (1981). The relationship of psychic healing and insight oriented treatment within an expressive framework. *Pratt Institute Creative Arts Therapy Review*, 2, 15–24.

Grubbs, G. (2016). The chakras in sandplay therapy. *Journal of Sandplay Therapy*, 25(2), 191–211.

Judith, A. (1987). *Wheels of life: A user's guide to the chakra system*. Llewellyn Worldwide.

Judith, A. (1996). *Eastern body, western mind: Psychology and the chakra system as a path to the self*. Celestial Arts.

Myss, C. (1996). *Anatomy of the Spirit*. Three Rivers Press.

Nelson, J. E. (1994). Madness or transcendence? Looking to the ancient East for a modern transpersonal diagnostic system. *ReVision*, 17(1), 14.

Nemri, K. (2004). Aiijii healing and how the chakras relate to disease and healing. *Proceedings (Academy of Religion & Physical Research)*, 36–42.

Rama, S., Ballentine, R., & Ajaya, S. (1976). *Yoga and psychotherapy: The evolution of consciousness*. Himalayan Publishers.

Rogers, M. E. (1970). *An introduction to the theoretical basis of nursing*. F. A. Davis.

Schneider, K. (2004). A qualitative and quantitative validation study of the assessment of the chakras through qualitative response (ACT-QR). California School of Professional Psychology, Fresno, CA.

5 Conceptualization and Change Processes

Physical and emotional pain serve as a call to action, a signal that some kind of change is required in order to thrive. Change can be scary, and is often paired with fears about losing control. However, authentic and effective change will always mean taking some level of risk, and requires a willingness to hold this uncertainty (Rama et al., 1976).

Learned Pain

Chronic pain and psychosomatic symptoms are now believed to be learned through maladaptive associations in the brain. The term psychophysiologic disorders is often used for these conditions to highlight the physical-neurologic component of this learning process. The symptom may be originating in the brain rather than the body, but the somatic experience of pain or discomfort is no less "real." Experiences of hunger and thirst are similarly produced in the brain yet clearly cause somatic distress.

Some of the latest medical treatments for psychosomatic conditions target *unlearning* pain through cognitive retraining and safety appraisal (e.g. Howard & Betzold, 2016). While these treatments are gaining empirical support, the language is misleading. In the field of psychology, we know that there is no such thing as "unlearning." Research has shown that behavioral responses can sometimes be extinguished, but then reappear after some time as passed ("spontaneous recovery") or as soon as a reinforcer is returned. Additionally, research on Relational Frame Theory (RFT) has demonstrated that humans learn through forming vast networks of relationships, which are often created outside of awareness and cannot be undone. As people repeatedly respond according to their relational frames, these pathways are strengthened and more likely to be used again for determining behavior.

Rather than thinking in terms of "unlearning", RFT and ACT suggest reframing the solution as building larger networks. This means adding more positive and helpful relational frames in order to overcome and minimize the impact of maladaptive relationships (Hayes, 2019). While previously learned pathways of stress cannot be removed, one can learn and strengthen a competing or alternative response. People can learn and

DOI: 10.4324/9781003251293-6

practice strategies to increase body awareness, reduce stressors, improve coping skills, and practice daily self-care; all of which create new relationships that allow them to develop more adaptive and values-based responses. Over time, these new pathways will be continuously strengthened and reinforced, while the previous pathways leading to somatic symptoms are weakened and become less important (rather than eliminated).

Notably, opposites are often a readily accessible relational frame. When people hear "cold," they think "hot." "Up" is associated with "down," and so on. This means that experiences of pain can be associated with relaxation, and vice versa, or that feelings of love and safety can trigger a memory of abuse (Hayes, 2019). These associations are normal, but can be distressing. It is essential that clinicians provide empathy and education regarding these cognitive processes, and continue to work towards building network relations that encourage the patient to move towards their values. If a relaxation technique seems to exacerbate their pain, try a more active somatic awareness technique (e.g. mindful walking) or engage the patient in scheduling a values-based activity (e.g. behavioral activation). Perhaps relaxation can be revisited later in treatment, but it is important to be continuously evaluating treatment based on the principles of contextual behaviorism and what "works" based on what helps the patient move in a values-based direction in that moment and within their context.

Drop the Rope

Both yoga and Acceptance and Commitment Therapy (ACT) recognize that efforts to control fundamentally cause internal conflict. ACT describes people as being caught in a tug-of-war with aspects of their mind (e.g. thought, feelings, memories). The only way to end this fruitless battle is to drop the rope, and acknowledge that control-and-eliminate strategies are not working. Once the struggle for control is given up, people can begin to move in a desired and meaningful direction. This is counterintuitive for most, as the larger culture and self-help media promote ideas of self-control and "fixing" one's life and problems. However, excessive effort only causes strain and tension. Self-threats or disparagement further increase distress (Hayes, 2019). Alternatively, relaxed detachment allows one to more easily reach their goals. This has been termed "passive volition", as opposed to strenuous "active volition" (Rama et al., 1976). The word "passive" in this sense, means objective and non-emotional.

Once unworkable strategies are given up, the problem is reframed in a way that opens individuals to identifying more adaptive and helpful strategies. The key turning point is the realization that (painful) experiences themselves do not cause symptoms, but rather one's *relationship* to their experiences (Hayes, 2019). Changing these relationships involves making room for all parts of experience inside awareness in order to focus on what matters most. This starts with fostering nonattachment and openness. In

Chakra-Organized Acceptance and Commitment Therapy (COACT) this is done with defusion and acceptance, while awareness skills are used to tune into one's relationship with their body and self. Flexible attention and relaxation exercises are used to observe the body and develop somatic awareness in order to learn from the body. Perspective-taking and self-as-context interventions develop self-awareness and self-integration, as the self-definition is expanded to encapsulate all experiences of the self. Lastly, identifying core values and engaging in committed action to pursue one's values improves functioning and life satisfaction.

Pathology from a Yoga Perspective

Holistic medicine suggests disease is that which interferes with an individual's basic wholeness, and that restoring wholeness promotes healing (Karagulla & van Gelder Kunz, 1989). This is primarily accomplished through removing barriers to the individual's self-heal-ing. In yoga psychology and humanistic psychotherapies, it is assumed that individuals have a natural tendency towards psychological growth and development. When this trajectory is disrupted, psychological dis-tress and symptomatology manifests. The clinician's goal is to help patients identify and understand what has interrupted their growth, and then resolve the problem in order to get "back on track." To suc-cessfully redirect, one must have an awareness and understanding of the "traps and pitfalls" that commonly disrupt self-discovery and growth (Rama et al., 1976). Certain harmful experiences, especially early in life, can lead people to develop maladaptive and rigid coping patterns that interfere with their ability to respond flexibly and adaptively to life experiences. Establishing healthy emotional and mental patterns are as essential in preventative health as a balanced diet and exercise (Karagulla & van Gelder Kunz, 1989). Barriers to health and healing can be defined in many different ways, such as incongruence (Client-Centered Therapy), energy imbalance (Yoga Psychology), or psycholo-gical inflexibility (ACT). Yet central to each of these theories is that experiences of trauma and stress can manifest as emotional, cognitive, physical, behavioral, and spiritual patterns that disrupt health and wellness.

Patanjali names five "kleshas" or "causes of misery" that narrow one's life and give way to experiences of emotional distress: 1) ignorance; 2) limited self-concept; 3) attachment; 4) aversion; and 5) fear of death (Hariharananda Aranya, 1963). Ignorance in this context refers to an attachment to a narrowly defined or limited reality. The kleshas are causes of suffering, as well as barriers to psychological and spiritual development (Rama et al., 1976). There is also some overlap between the kleshas, and all limit one's experience as a result of inflexible attachment.

Traumatic Stress and Chakras

Trauma and stress exposure can foster an orientation towards physical survival and self-preservation, which may come at the expense of mental and spiritual development. Studies expanding upon Felitti and colleagues' (1998) original adverse childhood experiences (ACEs) research further illuminated the context of psychophysiologic disorders and psychosomatic symptoms. These physical symptoms often result from coping strategies that are no longer adaptive for an individual's current environment or circumstances. When people bring awareness to how they have learned to respond as a result of trauma, they become free to choose alternative actions.

In humanistic language, trauma experiences that are suppressed or rejected create an incongruence between the individual's self-concept and experience. These discrepancies are painful and maintained by avoidance-based coping strategies. Chakra imbalance can be conceptualized as a form of incongruence: an aspect of the individual's experience is not in sync with another part. The chakra system encompasses psychological, physical, and spiritual components of the self, and discrepancies can exist in and between any of these domains. Imbalance in the chakra system may originate in an early life experience. However, energy disruption can also develop at any point in an individual's life in response to environmental, interpersonal, and situational factors; particularly those that are stressful. These energy blocks interfere with daily functioning by establishing or maintaining rigid maladaptive patterns of thoughts, actions, emotions, and physical sensations. In other words, chakra imbalance produces psychological inflexibility.

ACEs and other experiences of stress lead to painful emotions, which prompt experiential avoidance and the development of rule-based behavioral patterns in order to manage distress. These habits pull attention out of the present and limit the flexibility of actions. As adults, many find themselves stuck in inflexible response patterns that have outlived their usefulness, and at the expense of vitality and the ability to engage in life fully. In COACT, these consequences of psychological inflexibility are conceptualized as disconnection from one's body, true Self, and values; all of which produce symptoms of physical and psychological distress. Pathology, therefore, stems from impaired functioning, not vice versa (Stroshal et al., 2012). Symptoms are signals that one is misaligned from their true Self and values.

Trauma experiences further prompt coping strategies which sensitize individuals to information perceived as relevant for a particular purpose (e.g. threat-detection, self-preservation, building resources), while desensitizing them to other information. In this way, trauma and stress can create "tunnel-vision" or a limited perspective of the self and one's experiences organized around certain rules and conceptualized narratives. The *content* of these rules and stories vary according to how and where the traumatic experience disrupts the chakra system, while the *function* of these processes is held constant: pain avoidance. Trauma can lead to a preoccupation with control and fears about losing control, while actions that seek to gain or maintain control contribute to avoidant patterns that perpetuate symptomatic distress. Alternatively, responses that confront and make room for a traumatic event and related emotions in one's experience tend to reduce distress and improve functioning (French et al., 2008).

Applying Psychological Flexibility to the Chakras

ACT focuses not on challenging or controlling symptoms, but on changing their context. This means altering one's relationship with the symptom and experientially learning new ways of responding in order to enhance functioning and values-based action. From a functional contextual perspective, the six psychological flexibility skills are not meant to be practiced at all times or in all situations, but used when they improve functioning (McCracken & Vowels, 2014).

Medical literature on the treatment of chronic pain and psychosomatic conditions highlight the importance of increased emotional awareness, reduced experiential avoidance, changes in self-image (e.g. integration of experiences, recognition that the self is not determined by pain), relaxation skills, and self-care/values engagement (Clarke et al., 2019). Applying the psychological flexibility skills to the chakra system hits all of these targets. The COACT model engages both the physical and psycho-emotional aspects of the chakras, and promotes integration of the body, mind, and spirit in a way that restores energy congruence and life engagement. As there is no empirical definition or measure of chakra energy, COACT uses the psychological flexibility model to heal chakras by addressing the consequences of blocked energy: rigid attachments and avoidance-based habits contributing to disconnection from one's body, true Self, and values. Body avoidance and self avoidance/rejection both further facilitate emotional avoidance and alexithymia. Figure 5.1. demonstrates how a pattern of pain avoidance based on inflexible attachments and rules for controlling pain depletes chakra energy and causes symptomatic distress. Each box represents a factor that interferes with healthy chakra energy. Figure 5.2 highlights the role of psychological inflexibility processes in the depletion of chakra energy.

The content of a trauma experience and where it is processed and stored in the body influences where energy is most likely to be disrupted in the chakra system. The location of a prominent energy block then influences the physical and psycho-emotional symptoms an individual experiences. Many reporting psychosomatic symptoms are unaware of the psychological component, so using the location and quality of the physical symptom to extrapolate where energy flow is likely disrupted in the chakra system allows clinicians to quickly identify psychological themes that may be relevant to their condition. Specifically, identifying the chakra most involved in the symptom(s) allows for connecting the physical symptom to an emotional experience that may be manifesting somatically (e.g. fear, guilt, anger), how the patient's perspective

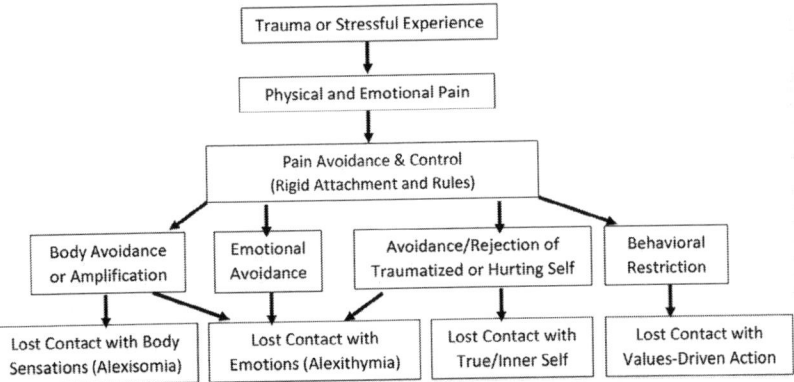

Figure 5.1. Chakra Energy Depletion

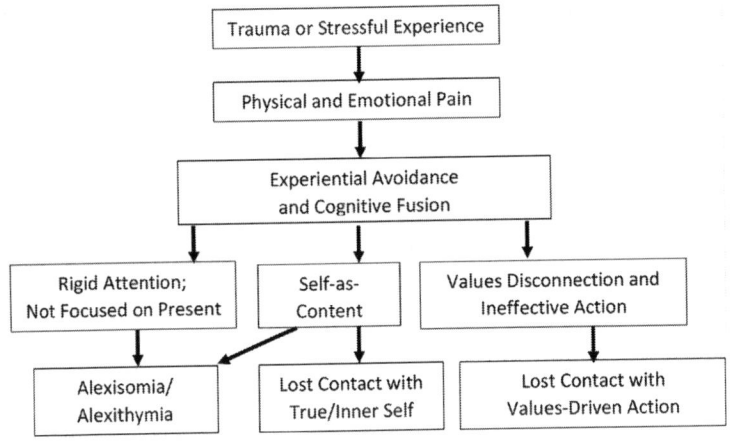

Figure 5.2. Inflexibility Processes and Chakra Energy

may be limited by a particular reference point (e.g. survival, pleasure, power), and which central values are not being expressed (e.g. family, independence, creativity). COACT uses the psychological flexibility skills to restore healthy energy through fostering general nonattachment (defusion and acceptance) and chakra-specific increases in somatic awareness (present attention skills), self-integration (perspective-taking and self-as-context skills), and values-based actions (values and committed action). Rather than focusing on symptom reduction, the goal of treatment is a complete experience of one's body, self, and life. Figure 5.3 provides a framework for how intervention seeks to restore balance and healthy energy through healing the consequences of disrupted chakras, and Figure 5.4 highlights the role of psychological flexibility skills.

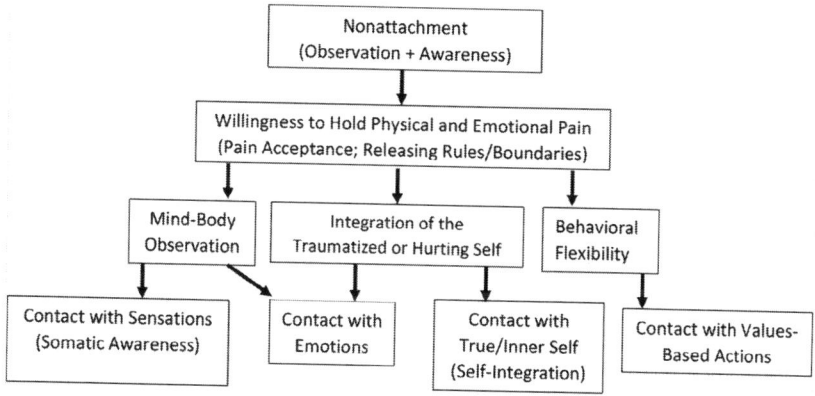

Figure 5.3. Chakra Energy Healing

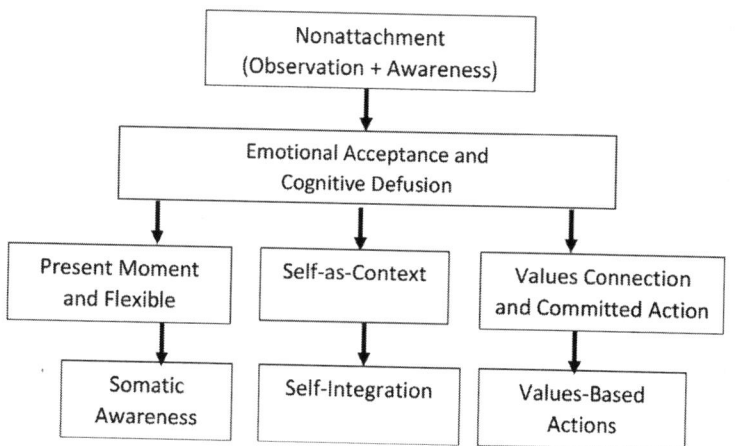

Figure 5.4. Flexibility Processes and Chakra Energy

In his *Principles of Behavior Modification* (Bandura, 1969), Albert Bandura recommended that therapy aim for the minimum change necessary to achieve a client's goals. There is no need for a complete reconstruction of the patient's sense of self or renovation of every habit. Instead, treatment targets areas most contributing to distress and where even subtle changes can ripple through the patient's life. Even a little energetic shift towards alignment can have a large functional impact.

Attachment vs. Nonattachment (Acceptance and Defusion)

The experience of attachment in yoga is conceptually similar to psychological inflexibility. Attachment functions much like rules that limit one's perspective, mental activity (e.g. thoughts and feelings), and ability to respond adaptively and flexibly to events. Experiences of extreme stress often elicit attachment patterns based on control and/or pain avoidance (e.g. numbing, distraction).

Attachment

Yoga systems view attachment, "the clinging to a familiar, and hence relatively secure concept of reality" as the ultimate barrier to self-realization and personal and spiritual growth, as well as the underlying source of all anxiety (Rama et al., 1976, p. 122). Attachment occurs when an individual is entangled with the contents of their mind and cannot observe themselves or a situation from an objective, unemotional stance. Attachment also results from experiences of pleasure or pain, such that individuals are motivated to seek experiences that produce pleasure, and are similarly motivated to avoid or suppress experiences which produce pain (Rama et al., 1976). Fusion and experiential avoidance are "two sides of the same coin" and hallmarks of psychological suffering (Strosahl & Robinson, 2008). However, avoidance-based strategies are not inherently dysfunctional, and prove adaptive in certain contexts. Avoidance becomes problematic when pain, whether emotional or physical, is viewed as an enemy to be eliminated (Hayes, 2019). The United States and other cultures tend to instill and perpetuate beliefs that negative emotions and thoughts are 1) pathological; 2) causally related to behavior; and 3) can be controlled by the same rules as external events (Hayes et al., 1996). All of these assumptions are false, yet many continue to apply these rules which maintain distress. These assumptions further reflect attachments to control and avoidance-based responses to pain.

Individuals can hold attachments to both internal and external activity. Mental attachments are called "sticky" thoughts in reference to how one becomes stuck to an experience due to emotional involvement (Hayes et al., 2012). When an internal event elicits a strong painful reaction, it pulls attention away from the moment and perpetuates restricted response patterns based on resolving or removing the painful feeling. In yoga, these sticky attachments are viewed as being "charged with energy" (Rama et al., 1976, p. 127). These charged mental events motivate impulsive and emotional action, which strengthens their energetic hold. It is said that the experience becomes "weighted with more karma" (Rama et al., 1976, p. 127), each time the mental event determines a behavioral response.

Basic learning theory similarly informs that a relationship between two events is strengthened when they occur together multiple times. Even activities meant to distract can come to be associated with the very pain or distress the individual is seeking to avoid through repeated pairings (i.e. classical conditioning), and the removal of distress caused by avoidance (i.e. negative reinforcement). As the relational frame network for pain grows, the individual has to spend more time and energy trying to eliminate pain. However, efforts to control painful mental events tend to only increase their salience. Much like Hercules battling the Hydra, the pain multiplies with each attempt to remove it. This attachment to control-avoid strategies narrowly restricts one's life space and experience.

Alexithymia and Pain Avoidance

Another consequence of trauma is an experiential disconnection from the mind and/or body that disrupts the inner communication system. This causes people to misread physiological and emotional cues, including important danger cues. Further, when symptoms of distress are viewed as problematic, control-avoid strategies are implemented to "kill the messenger" and destroy natural alarm systems in the mind and body (Stroshal et al., 2012). Living without these signals is like wearing "emotional blinders" (Hayes, 2019, p. 195), and increases the likelihood of revictimization (Fiorillo et al., 2013). Difficulties with emotional awareness can also result from growing-up in emotionally-controlled families or cultures, where emotions are generally unexpressed or poorly communicated.

Problems with interpreting emotional and physiological cues can manifest as alexithymia and alexisomia. Alexithymia is a deficit in experiencing and describing emotions, while alexisomia is the inability to observe physiological sensations (Bakal, 1999). Mental rigidity consists of alexithymia and experiential avoidance (Hayes, 2019). The term alexithymia was first used in a discussion of characteristics found in patients with psychosomatic symptoms (Sifneos, 1973). This skill deficit has been linked to physical symptoms, negative subjective reports of health, and increased risk of death due to accident, injury, or violence (Kauhanen et al., 1996). Poor awareness of internal processes may interfere with taking preventative action, seeking medical treatment when needed, and accurately reporting symptoms to healthcare professionals (Bakal, 1999). However, teaching patients to be more emotionally and somatically self-aware can help reduce the negative health impacts of alexithymia and alexisomia.

Nonattachment

The yoga psychology meaning of nonattachment is a state of openness where one is able to reflect on objects and experiences as they are, without having their perspective narrowed by emotions, rule-based thinking, or motivations to move towards or away certain outcomes. Nonattachment is a state of defusion and acceptance, making room for all experiences. From a detached perspective, internal events are interpreted as transient, natural, and not inherently meaningful. A thought is just a thought, a feeling just a feeling. The content of thoughts, feelings, or sensations does not determine their usefulness, but rather how these experiences help or hurt an individual in pursuing their values. Nonattachment releases the emotional weight tied to an experience, allowing the energy to dissipate and lose its power.

Defusion involves de-literalizing the impact of mental content. Distress often occurs when people react to private events as if they imply something about the Self or require action, thus prompting efforts to regulate or control these experiences. Through defusion individuals learn to let go of rule-based contingencies guiding both private and external action, and alternatively select actions based on experiential consequences. The human mind, with its expertise in symbolic thought and propensity for problem-solving, is often operating according to rule-based contingencies and remarkably poor at letting go of these fixations. Once someone learns a rule for behavior, they tend to adhere to that rule even when experience demonstrates this rule is ineffective. Instead of letting go of an ineffective strategy, humans may even double-down, justify their rule-driven strategy with additional rules, and/or blame their failure on external factors (Hayes, 2019). Growing up you may have heard, "If at first you don't succeed, try, try again." This exemplifies how humans are taught from the beginning of life to follow rules, even over experience.

Acceptance is a state of willingness, and allowing one's experience to be what it is. This does not mean liking or enjoying the experience, but simply being willing to have it. ACT clinicians may use the axiom, "If you don't want it, you have it," to demonstrate that unwillingness to hold a particular experience is a perfect way to continue struggling with it. Acceptance is giving up this struggle with experience in order to focus on meaningful action. Individuals need contact with their painful experiences in order to acknowledge and learn from them. Painful events are often one's greatest teachers for learning how to grow and adapt in pursuit of their values. Without this contact, people are disconnected not only from information that can help them move in a more meaningful direction, but also information that helps prevent them from making the same mistakes. Pain highlights where people are invested, and nonattachment allows one to observe this pain in order to better understand what is needed to heal. Two key components of pain acceptance are 1) willingness to experience pain; and, 2) engaging in values-based activities even when pain is present (McCracken et al., 2004).

Pain Acceptance and Releasing Attachments

Letting go of attachments requires a complete re-evaluation of what has been defined as desirable and undesirable, and then dispassionately releasing both. As attachments are released, greater variability opens up and one can choose responses based on values rather than rules of control or avoidance. It is important to understand the rules of a patient's pain management, as these may be the very same habits that are maintaining distress. What do they do when they first notice the pain? Do they take pain relieving medication? Do they sit or lay down and try to rest, or do they try to "fight through" the pain? What situations or movements do they avoid? What do they "have to do" in order to prevent flare ups or worsening pain? Many patients with psychosomatic symptoms, especially those that have had their symptom for many years, will have very specific and rigid routines established. The thought of doing something different may be extremely anxiety provoking, as they are certain any deviation from their usual habits will lead to unbearable pain. This is a great opportunity for exploring workability and developing a sense of creative hopelessness. Is their current routine really *working* for them? What are the short-term and long-term consequences? What values or experiences have they had to give up? This can be a challenging and emotional process for the patient as they come to realize their current strategies and attachments are part of the problem.

Body Avoidance & Amplification vs. Somatic Awareness (Present Attention)

Stress impacts every level of experience, from the psyche to the cells. Psychosomatic symptoms are often the body's reaction to an emotional or situational stressor that has occurred outside a person's awareness. An individual may only notice the physiological response when it becomes severe enough to cause distress, and distress is enhanced by a lack of understanding regarding the symptoms' cause (Bakal, 1999). Developing somatic awareness, therefore, serves to bring these physiologic experiences into conscious awareness to enhance understanding and response selection.

Gathering information from the body requires the ability to observe and be present with physiologic sensations with the same detached, voluntary focus needed to observe the mind. Body sensations are typically vague, and difficult to localize or measure. Thus, it requires active and conscious attention in order to be able to use this information to improve health. Noticing pain, discomfort, or unusual sensations in the body is usually done readily and without conscious effort (e.g., racing heart, shortness of breath), while bringing awareness to more routine, non-emotional body sensations (e.g., relaxed heart rate) requires more deliberate attention. Further, most people are not very accurate in reading or interpreting their physiological sensations, although they can refine this skill with training and practice (Bakal, 1999). Present moment and flexible attention skills taught in ACT help develop this awareness, as well as various mind-body and relaxation techniques such as mindfulness, yoga stretching, breathing exercises, muscle relaxation, and imagery.

Body Avoidance

In order to divert all attention to self-preservation during times of stress, people often tune-out other messages from the mind and body. Over time, they may become unable to tune back in. Developing a habit of body avoidance and chronic pain symptoms after physical trauma exposure is common (Leserman et al., 1996). Individuals learn to separate their awareness from the body in order to survive a threatening situation and/or cope with the repercussions (e.g. injuries, physical damage). This is a remarkable way the mind and body demonstrate resilience, but is not adaptive in the long-term. When individuals disconnect from the pain in the body, they also lose contact with the information and wisdom the body has to offer. Bodily sensations are also a key component of emotions, such that attending to somatic cues is important for labeling and understanding emotional experiences.

Identification of distress in the body tends to enhance a desire to avoid somatic experiences, which maintains and increases pain over time. Fear, confusion, and frustration associated with physical pain may further prompt individuals to turn attention away from the problem. It is common for individuals to depersonalize or objectify their pain, such as referring to the symptom or the affected part of the body as "it" (Bakal, 1999). Examples include statements like, "Why is it happening to me?", "It won't leave me alone!", and "I just want to get rid of it." In this way, the symptom is often externalized as something outside of the patient's experience, rather than a part of it.

Body Amplification and Cognitive Misattribution of Physical Sensations

Two other mechanisms of somatization are body amplification and cognitive misattribution (Bakal, 1999). Body amplification refers to the tendency to exaggerate or exhibit a heightened sensitivity to physiologic sensations that others may experience as benign. This is commonly associated with anxiety, where an individual demonstrates hypervigilance to body sensations, a propensity for attending to mild or unusual sensations, and a tendency for interpreting these sensations as pathological (Bakal, 1999). However, the cognitive biases associated with both anxiety and depression influence reports of somatic symptoms. Individuals with anxiety tend to experience heightened vigilance which increases their in-the-moment attention to mild and moderate changes in physiological sensations. Those with depression tend to experience more rumination and a recall bias whereby their recall of previously experienced somatic symptoms is negatively exaggerated. Thus, anxiety is associated with an inflated report of current physical symptoms, while depression is associated with inflated recall of past physical symptoms (Suls & Howren, 2012).

Other research suggests that increased body awareness does not necessarily contribute to pathology, but that body awareness from the perspective of being ill does (Hansell & Mechanic, 1991). From a perspective of illness attribution, people select and attend to information that corroborates this assumption, while missing opportunities for other interpretations or therapeutic action. Once convinced there is a biomedical disease causing the symptom, the individual is likely to believe the symptom is outside their control and can only be treated with medical intervention (e.g. medication, surgery). This attribution can be difficult to alter, but must be challenged in order for a patient to believe their personal actions can improve their symptoms (Bakal, 1999). Importantly, cognitive misattributions are not mutually exclusive with physiologic pathology. For example, a patient may be preoccupied with the belief that gastro-intestinal symptoms are indicative of ulcers when the actual physiologic cause is a mild food intolerance. Emotional distress and cultural beliefs play a critical role in how individuals interpret and experience their symptoms.

Somatic Awareness

COACT aims to facilitate communication between the mind and body (i.e. mind-body congruence) through the development of somatic awareness. Bodies constantly work to achieve and maintain homeostasis and balance, and somatic experiences motivate behavior through an association with emotions and meaning-making processes. Somatic awareness is the ability to observe physiological sensations, connect these sensations with emotions, and intuitively listen to the body to inform self-care activities. Everyone has the capacity for somatic awareness, and for tuning into their body's natural wisdom for health and healing (Bakal, 1999). Somatic awareness encourages individuals to be curious about the body's communication and need expression. Noticing shoulder tension or restricted breathing, for example, may indicate stress or anxiety and a need for relaxation. Early detection allows for quicker and more efficient responses to restore health. It is common for individuals with chronic pain to actually increase body tension when they first notice symptoms as they brace themselves for worsening pain or a "flare-up." This tends to make the symptoms worse and contributes to a sense of helplessness, as if nothing can be done but prepare for the pain. With increased body awareness, individuals can observe the sensations guiding behavior, and make conscious decisions to regulate these sensations for optimized health and wellbeing. Strategies based on control or avoidance are contrary to somatic awareness, while techniques that foster somatic awareness include diaphragmatic breathing, yoga stretching, muscle relaxation, and leisure activities (e.g. reading, listening to music). Essentially all self-regulating techniques and methods of tracking expansion and contraction in the body help develop somatic awareness (Bakal, 1999). Further, when clinicians and patients feel stuck, centering on somatic awareness and listening to the body can help orient the patient and guide next steps.

Chakras and Somatic Awareness

The chakra system provides a framework for practicing targeted somatic awareness. Based on where pain or symptoms are occurring in the body, somatic awareness techniques can be used to focus attention on that chakra in order to access its wisdom, learn from the body, and heal that chakra's

Table 5.1 Chakras and Somatic Symptoms

Root	Sacral	Solar Plexus	Heart	Throat	Brow
Lower back, feet, ankle, or knee; fatigue, immune conditions	Genito-pelvic area hips, bladder, kidney, spleen, reproductive system	Abdomen, stomach/GI tract (e.g. nausea, gastritis), middle spine, pancreas, liver	Chest, upper back, shoulder, arm, diaphragm/rib area, lungs (dyspnea, hyperventilation, asthma/allergies), accelerated heart rate	Throat, mouth, neck pain, feelings of choking or difficulty swallowing, esophagitis	Head/face-Migraines, headaches, dizziness, insomnia, sensory dysfunction, sinusitis, seizures

energy. Table 5.1 is a quick reference for body areas and somatic symptoms primarily associated with each chakra.

Limited or Conceptualized Self vs. Transcendent Self and Self-Integration (Self-as-Context)

Many therapies aim to help individuals develop an accurate and stable sense of self. The development of self is a process that can begin in therapy, but will continue throughout the lifetime. A key role of therapy is facilitating the initial self-direction. Client-centered therapy helps clients recognize and confront incongruence between the self-concept and experience, re-examine the self, and modify their self-concept to integrate aspects of their experience. These changes may be modest or robust, but signify a new direction for the self. As the individual's self-perceptions change, their behavior and external perceptions change too. With a modified and more authentic sense of self, individuals choose different actions and see the world differently (Rogers, 1951). ACT uses perspective-taking and self-as-context skills to facilitate contact with the transcendent self and develop a flexible self-concept.

Limited and Conceptualized Self

The self interprets information received through the senses and attributes meaning to experiences. When the sense of self is attached to an external object or conceptualized narrative, the mind takes over orienting the individual in their environment. With the mind in command, people evaluate rather than experience, and analyze rather than bring awareness to. Many challenges result from overidentifying with the mind's perspective. The mind is skilled at identifying and fixing problems, and will turn this problem-solving ability inward, selecting aspects of the self to be "fixed" or even removed. This mind is not an enemy to the self, but a powerful and useful tool meant to be used by the self. When individuals fuse with their mind, they lose their ability to observe and discriminate their mental processes (Rama et al., 1976). In this way, individuals may fuse their self-concept with the contents of their mind (e.g. thoughts, feelings, memories). ACT labels this "self-as-content" (Hayes et al., 2012). The self-concept is then limited by attachments which narrow one's perspective, such as self-stories and conceptualized versions of the self (e.g. idealized self, pain-free self). Fusion with a conceptualized self also leads to poor contact with the transcendent or "true" Self and one's central values.

Humans' ability with symbolic language contributes to strong attachments as individuals develop self-stories that are experienced as real. Loss of the conceptualized self may produce anxiety or fear, as releasing this narrative may feel like losing one's self. At the extreme, the idea of letting go of the conceptualized self could feel like death (Rama et al., 1976). Further, when one is fused with a particular identity or self-concept, they become motivated to maintain this persona. People lose the ability to observe their own responses and experiences objectively as they cling to information that supports the desired narrative and reject that which contradicts it. They may lie to defend this conceptualized self-image or end relationships with those who do not confirm their self-perception. Whether the conceptualized self is positive or negative is of less importance than how rigidly it determines one's self-concept (Hayes, 2019).

Self-Integration

Yoga psychology views psychological growth as the process of bringing awareness to aspects of the self believed to be intolerable or unacceptable, and then allowing them to be integrated into the whole (Rama et al., 1976). Self-integration therefore refers to systematically observing the limitations in the current self-concept and then expanding the sense of self to make room for more of one's true experience. This first requires a practice of self-observation, and an attitude of willingness to hold all experiences, even pain. Training the body to relax and reduce external distractions helps with observing one's self and mental activities. This stillness allows memories, sensations, and feelings typically outside one's awareness to come to the surface. Introspection develops self-awareness and a calm, objective, and honest evaluation of one's current self, including recognizing the limits of the existing "I." One can then give up the frenzied and frantic struggles of the limited self, such as pursuits of perfection or pain control (Rama et al., 1976). When limitations are acknowledged, one can explore and discover where they are stuck and where they can make room or expand the self-concept.

Developing a flexible and adaptive self-definition is part of Patanjali's idea of living in awareness rather than ignorance (Remski, 2012). ACT also emphasizes the need for a flexible self-concept in order to move beyond the rigid boundaries that limit the full experience of the self. To detach from limited self-conceptualizations, individuals need to defuse from the self-judgments and expectations that may stem from oneself or others, and create acceptance for parts of the self that have been rejected or dismissed. This includes releasing maladaptive narratives in order to connect with the stable and transcendent self and integrate all aspects of the self, including the "traumatized" or hurting parts of the self.

Interventions to increase psychological flexibility (i.e. ACT) have been used to enhance malleability of self-concept in order to improve functioning and values-based action. Perspective taking is the ACT process that specifically addresses expanding one's self-definition, and includes self-as-process and self-as-context. Self-as-context refers to viewing the true Self as a separate container for one's experiences, while self-as-process is the awareness of one's ongoing experiencing process (Hayes et al., 2012). Self-as-context skills can be used to detach from a sense of self defined by one's pain experience (fusion with or avoidance of) and flexibly contextualize the meaning of one's pain. This entails observing pain sensations with emotional detachment and developing an awareness of pain as a sensation in the body without inherent meaning about one's self, goals, or values.

Chakras and Self-Integration

Yoga psychology and the chakra system offer an organization of the self that allows for targeted intervention. Each chakra is associated with particular qualities or attributes of the self. Rejection of these selves produces energy disruption, while perspective-taking strategies can be applied to connect with these different self-perspectives. As an example, an individual may develop a self-story that they no longer experience "weak" emotions and pour their energy into their work as a distraction from the pain of a romantic breakup. This pain reflects concerns of the sacral chakra, so making contact with emotional and playful aspects of the self may help restore balance and reduce distress.

Each chakra is further associated with an emotional experience of the self that can also be distorted or denied due to trauma/stress. Emotional distress exacerbates physical pain or discomfort, and emotional suppression contributes to increased pain sensitivity and avoidance (Burns et al., 2008). Alternatively, pain acceptance can help resolve both emotional and somatic symptoms. When difficult emotions are rejected, the part of the self who experiences this emotion is rejected too. Therefore, part of making room for all of the self is making room for all emotions, including those that are painful. The observing perspective can help individuals hold these feelings without becoming entangled in them. Chakra healing is promoted by allowing these emotions to enter awareness and be accepted into one's experience by expanding the self-concept and developing flexible perspective-taking skills. Individuals try to relate to the self that is hurting, see through their eyes, and accept this self and their pain. Table 5.2 summarizes the self-perspectives and emotions associated with each chakra.

Table 5.2. Chakras and Self-Perspectives

	Root	Sacral	Solar Plexus	Heart	Throat	Brow	Crown
Self-Perspective	Physical & Grounded	Emotional & Playful	Powerful & Responsible	Compassionate & Social	Honest & Contributing	Curious & Reflective	Universal & Transpersonal
Emotion	Fear	Guilt/ Blame	Shame/ Anger	Jealousy/ Resentment & Grief	Doubt/ Judgment	Depression/ Despair	Existential Angst

Behavioral Restriction vs. Values-Based Action (Values and Committed Action)

Participating in activities that are self-affirming, prosocial, and healthy improves general wellbeing and fosters connection with the self and body through caring for one's mental and physical health. Thoughts, feelings, and other internal material are primarily of clinical interest in how they guide an individual's behavioral responses. Changes in behavior can further produce changes in emotional and cognitive experiences. All behaviors reflect an individual's meaningful efforts to adapt to their environment. As an individual develops insight, they learn to consciously alter their behaviors to choose actions that are more responsible and aligned with their true Self (Rogers, 1951).

Behavioral Restriction

Experiences of trauma can trigger survival instincts and the most basic psychological behavioral patterns. These automatic responses place one's values on the back burner in order to prioritize more immediate concerns, such as survival or self-preservation. Trauma experiences tend to elicit automatic habits of responding that help people survive stressful situations, but are no longer adaptive or functionally workable once the stressor has passed. Muscle tension in the body or emotional suppression, for example, help protect in the short-term but can cause harmful consequences if prolonged. Restricted behavioral patterns learned from trauma and stress have to be consciously challenged as individuals work to discover whether their actions are aligned with their core values.

Attachments and avoidance-based strategies perpetuate a sense of disconnection. Steven Hayes suggests ineffective action stems from a misdirected yearning for meaning, which occurs primarily for four reasons: 1) a lack of trust in oneself to make appropriate choices; 2) concern that one's values are in contrast to societal or cultural norms; 3) fusion with a conceptualized self-image; and 4) pain avoidance. The immediate relief or gratification that occurs during pain avoidance gets mistaken for meaning, and people get stuck in a rigid or rule-based behavioral pattern in pursuit of these superficial satisfactions and external validation (Hayes, 2019). In other words, they become controlled by attachments rather than values.

Values-Based Action

Discussing values in the early part of treatment helps establish a desired direction. Ask the patient, "What would you be doing if you did not have pain?" or "What would you want to do if your pain was not a barrier?" Questions like this help to reveal who and what is most important to them. The removal of pain is not always an option, and is not the goal of treatment. Individuals may have to accept parts of their pain in order to pursue their values. Consider the options to have pain and attend your daughter's wedding, or to have pain and *not* attend your daughter's wedding, which do you want to do? It is also important to help the patient experiment with small steps that begin to create space for what they have been avoiding (physical sensations, emotions, self-awareness) in order to pursue values-based actions.

Chakras and Committed Action

ACT literature references many life domains that can guide values, including: family, friends, work, fun/recreation, community, environment, self-care, physical health, spirituality, and education. In identifying values individuals may consider what they really want in each of these domains, which are most important, and how they want to engage with each aspect of life. Encourage patients to identify any barriers, both internal and external, to values-based behavior, and consider how one can respond in order to continue moving in a values-based direction. Practicing openness and nonattachment (i.e. defusion and acceptance) inspires more effective coping with these challenges. Each chakra governs a different set of values, although some values may be supported by more than one chakra. Table 5.3 provides a few examples of values associated with each chakra. However, this list is not exhaustive.

Personality Attributes and Coping Styles

Certain personality and emotionality characteristics have been associated with greater reports of psychosomatic symptoms. This group of traits has been termed "Type C coping", and broadly reflects an orientation towards self-sacrifice and seeking to please others, paying attention to everyone except themselves (Bakal, 1999). These individuals may be extremely compassionate towards others while highly self-critical and preoccupied with being a "good" person (Clarke et al., 2019). They tend to be cooperative, responsible, passive and appeasing, externally-focused, and

Table 5.3 Chakras and Values

Root	Sacral	Solar Plexus	Heart	Throat	Brow
Family, Group Belonging, Health, Nature, Physical Activity, Order, Safety, Stability Trust, Self-Care	Adventure, Beauty, Control, Excitement/ Fun, Humor, Pleasure, Romance, Sensuality, Sexuality, Self-Gratification	Assertiveness, Challenge, Courage, Independence, Persistence, Power, Responsibility, Self-Esteem, Skillfulness, Self-Development	Compassion, Empathy, Equality, Forgiveness, Generosity, Intimacy, Kindness, Love, Relationships, Self-Acceptance	Authenticity, Community Service, Contribution, Creativity, Honesty, Humility, Industry, Integrity, Justice, Self-Expression	Clarity, Curiosity, Gratitude, Imagination, Knowledge, Mindfulness, Open-Mindedness, Wisdom, Spirituality, Self-Awareness

emotionally-controlled. It is also common for people in this population to exhibit Type A traits, such as perfectionism, a high need for accomplishment and success, and a tendency to overextend themselves and always keep busy. In order to keep up with personal responsibilities and external expectations, these individuals often avoid or deny both emotional and physical experiences that might challenge their need for composure and control.

As psychosomatic symptoms appear to be more related to coping style and psychosocial factors than organic disease processes, treatment often emphasizes changes in coping. One such shift is at the cognitive level, which includes one's attributions and perceived level of control of their symptom. For example, beliefs that the symptom is an indicator of serious illness tend to be associated with feelings of hopelessness, helplessness, and passive coping strategies. Beliefs that the symptom is a learning opportunity or challenge to be managed and overcome, rather, tend to be associated with feelings of empowerment, resilience, and active coping strategies (Bakal, 1999). Another shift is at the emotional level, where an individual learns to identify and express the feelings they tend to reject, ignore, or bottle up (e.g., anger, fear, grief, shame, guilt). Their symptoms may be due to a somatic expression of these painful emotions, and verbal or written expression has been associated with symptom relief. A third shift is behavioral and involves developing self-care skills (Clarke et al., 2019).

References

Ajaya, S. (1976). *Yoga psychology: A practical guide to mediation.* The Himalayan International Institute of Yoga Science and Philosophy of the U.S.A.

Bakal, D. (1999). *Minding the body: Clinical uses of somatic awareness.* Guilford.

Bandura, A. (1969). *Principles of behavior modification.* Holt, Rinehart and Winston.

Burns, J.W., Quartana, P., Gilliam, W., Gray, E., Matsuura, J., Nappi, C., Wolfe, B., & Lofland, K. (2008). Effects of angry suppression on pain sensitivity and pain behaviors among chronic pain patients: Evaluation of an ironic process model. *Health Psychology*, 27, 645–652.

Clarke, D. D., Schubiner, H., Clark-Smith, M., & Abbass, A. (Eds.) (2019). *Psychophysiologic disorders: Trauma informed, interprofessional diagnosis and treatment.* Psychophysiologic Disorders Association.

Felitti, V. J., Anda, R. F., Nordenberg, D., Williamson, D. F., Spitz, A. M., Edwards, V., Koss, M. P., & Marks, J. S. (1998). Relationship of childhood abuse and household dysfunction to many of the leading causes of death in adults. The adverse childhood experiences (ACE) study. *American Journal of Preventive Medicine*, 14(4), 245–258.

Fiorillo, D., Papa, A., & Follette, V. M. (2013). The relationship between child physical abuse and victimization in dating relationships: The role of experiential avoidance. *Psychological Trauma: Theory, Research, Practice, and Policy*, 5(6), 562–569.

French, F. J., Mennin, D. S., Smith, R. L., et al. (2008). The impact of pretrauma analogue GAD and posttraumatic emotional reactivity following exposure to the September 11 terrorist attacks: A longitudinal study. *Behavior Therapy*, 39, 262–276.

Hansell, S., & Mechanic, D. (1991). Body awareness and self-assessed health among older adults. *Journal of Aging and Health*, 3, 473–492.

Hariharananda Aranya, S. (1963). *Yoga philosophy of Patanjali*. University of Calcutta.

Hayes, S. C. (2019). *A liberated mind: How to pivot toward what matters*. Avery.

Hayes, S. C., Strosahl, K. D. & Wilson, K. G. (2012). *Acceptance and commitment therapy: The process and practice of mindful change* (2nd ed.). Guilford.

Hayes, S. C. , Wilson, K. G., Strosahl, K., Gifford, E. V., & Follette, V. M. (1996). Experiential avoidance and behavioral disorders: A functional dimensional approach to diagnosis and treatment. *Journal of Consulting and Clinical Psychology*, 64, 1152–1168.

Howard, H., & Betzold, M. (2016). *Unlearn your pain* (3rd ed.). Mind Body Publishing.

Karagulla, S., & van Gelder Kunz, D. (1989). *The chakras and the human energy field.* Quest Books.

Kauhanen, J., Kaplan, G. A., Cohen, R. D., Julkunen, J., & Salonen, J. T. (1996). Alexithymia and risk of death in middle-aged men. *Journal of Psychosomatic Research*, 41(6), 541–549.

Leserman, J., Drossman, D. A., Li, Z., Toomey, T. C., Nachman, G., & Glogau, L. (1996). Sexual and physical abuse history in gastroenterology practice: How types of abuse impact health status. *Psychosomatic Medicine*, 58, 4–15.

McCracken, L. M., & Vowels, K. E. (2014). Acceptance and commitment therapy and mindfulness for chronic pain: Model, process, and progress. *American Psychologist*, 69 (2), 178–187.

McCracken, L. M., Vowels, K. E., & Eccleston, C. (2004). Acceptance of chronic pain: Component analysis and a revised assessment method. *Pain*, 107(1–2), 159–166.

Rama, S., Ballentine, R., & Ajaya, S. (1976). *Yoga and psychotherapy: The evolution of consciousness*. Himalayan Publishers.

Remski, M. (2012). *Threads of yoga: A remix of patañjali's sutras, with commentary and reverie*. Bookbaby.

Rogers, C. R. (1951). *Client-centered therapy: It's current practice, implications, and theory*. Houghton Mifflin.

Sifneos, P. E. (1973). The prevalence of 'alexithymic' characteristics in psychosomatic patients. *Psychotherapy and Psychosomatics*, 22, 255–262.

Strosahl, K., & Robinson, P. J. (2008). *The mindfulness and acceptance workbook for depression: Using acceptance and commitment therapy to move through depression and create a life worth living*. New Harbinger.

Strosahl, K., Robinson, P., & Gustavsson, T. (2012). *Brief interventions for radical change: Principles & practice of focused acceptance & commitment therapy*. New Harbinger.

Suls, J., & Howren, M. B. (2012). Understanding the physical-symptom experience: The distinctive contributions of anxiety and depression. *Current Directions in Psychological Science*, 21(2), 129–134.

6 Treatment Orientation
Evaluation and Fostering Nonattachment

The first part of this chapter outlines how clinicians can complete an evaluation in order to create an effective conceptualization and treatment plan. Utilizing the chakra model as a guide, the clinician will begin to identify where the patient is disconnected from their body, their self, and their values. The second half of this chapter will introduce strategies for developing nonattachment through acceptance and defusion techniques.

Evaluation

An evaluation of the patient's current symptoms and relevant history is needed to initiate treatment. During this evaluation, the clinician particularly listens for physical symptoms, self-perceptions, painful emotions, patterns of avoidance, and values; all of which are relevant for identifying themes of chakra dysfunction. A summary tool of the evaluation components (Appendix A) is provided to assist clinicians in this evaluation. During the evaluation, the clinician introduces the format and structure of therapy, and collaborates with the patient to prioritize problems and discuss treatment goals.

Life Context: Contextual Interview

An evaluation of psychosomatic symptoms begins with a contextual interview (Robinson, 2020). The contextual interview format was developed alongside Focused Acceptance and Commitment Therapy (FACT; Strosahl et al., 2012) in order to quickly and effectively capture a patient's life and health context. There are four domains in the contextual interview: Love, Work, Play, and Health. Example questions within each domain are provided below. Other life domains for inquiry may include religion/spiritual background, strengths, and values.

1 Love: *Who do you live with? How is your relationship with each person in the home? What is your relationship status? How long have you been partnered/*

DOI: 10.4324/9781003251293-7

married? *How are your relationships with family/friends? Who are the most important people in your life?*

2   Work/School: *What do you do for work? Full-time or part-time? Are you in school? Do you enjoy your work/school? How is your work-life balance?*

3   Play: *What do you do for fun or relaxation? Do you have any hobbies? What do you do that is just for you?*

4   Health: *Do you have difficulty falling or staying asleep? How many hours of sleep/night do you get? How is your energy level during the day? Any changes in your diet/appetite? How many meals do you eat? Do you regularly exercise or engage in physical activity? Do you smoke or use other tobacco/nicotine products? How much? Caffeine? Alcohol? Other substances?*

Problem Context

The most salient symptom for the patient and the reason they are seeking treatment is likely their physical pain or somatic distress. However, if a clinician is interested in screening for psychophysiological stress reactions, the Patient Health Questionnaire-15 (PHQ-15; Kroenke et al., 2002) can be used to assess for fifteen different somatic symptoms (e.g. back pain, nausea, chest pain, stomach pain, arm/leg pain, shortness of breath, sexual discomfort). To better understand the patient's symptom experience and context, the clinician inquires about the symptoms' timing, trajectory, and triggers ("3 Ts", Robinson, 2020).

1   Timing: *When did the pain/symptom start? Was anything else significant happening at that time? Was the onset gradual or acute?*

2   Trajectory: *How has the pain/symptom been present over time? Has it been getting progressively worse, fluctuating, or improving? Are there times when the symptom is not present?*

3   Triggers: *What seems to make the pain/symptom worse? Are there any factors that seem to increase the frequency, intensity, or duration of the symptom?*

In determining whether a symptom is related to a psychophysiologic condition, a clinician assesses the chronology of pain and its context, looking for signs that the pain is inconsistent with structural damage. The Psychophysiologic Disorders Association (PPDA; Clarke et al., 2019) offers the acronym "FIT" (Functional, Inconsistent, Triggered) to help clinicians rule-out organic causes of symptoms, although medical consultation remains imperative. See the "FIT" Test (Appendix B) for a list of symptom qualities that suggest a psychophysiologic condition is present. Psychophysiologic disorders can be comorbid with structural damage, but occur when the subjective symptomatic experience is more severe or incongruent with symptoms caused by the physical anomaly alone.

Stress Evaluation

After gathering general information about the patient and their presenting problem, it is important to learn more about their experiences of stress or trauma. Patients may have already reported some of these experiences during the contextual interview, or the clinician may need to inquire further. Ask about any current or ongoing stressors, and invite the patient to rate their current stress on a scale of 0 to 10 (0 indicating no stress and 10 indicating extremely high levels of stress). Clinicians also assess self-care, stress management, and coping skills (Clarke et al., 2019).

One way to assess historical stress is with the Adverse Childhood Experiences (ACE) Questionnaire first used by Felitti and colleagues (1998). This questionnaire asks individuals to indicate whether or not they experienced ten different stressful events (ACEs) prior to age 18. The categories include experiences of physical and emotional neglect; physical, emotional, and sexual abuse; domestic violence; separation from a parent due to death, divorce, or abandonment; and a family member's incarceration, mental illness, or substance abuse. As these ten items do not cover all potential experiences of stress in childhood, many healthcare professionals have opted for more inclusive measures and screening tools. One is the Life Events Checklist (LEC-5; Weathers et al., 2013), which lists 17 stressful events, including an item for "any other stressful event or experience." Individuals are asked whether they personally experienced, witnessed, or learned about an incident of each event, as well as whether this exposure was part of their job. The Trauma History Questionnaire (THQ; Hooper et al., 2011) similarly provides 24 examples of stressful events, and asks individuals to indicate which they have experienced, if the exposure was repeated/frequency of exposure, and at what age they experienced each event.

David Clarke, MD, president of the Psychophysiologic Disorders Association (PPDA), created the Hidden Stress Screening Test (Clarke, n.d.) to quickly and broadly inquire about key stress symptoms. The screener asks patients to rate the amount of stress they have experienced recently, how often they neglect their own needs and self-care in order to prioritize caring for others, and how they would feel if they learned that a child they care about was experiencing the same childhood they had. This last question aims to overcome the potential tendency to downplay or minimize one's own painful experiences. Reports of feeling very sad or angry in response are interpreted as the patient likely having experienced ACEs. Alternatively, the clinician could ask the patient to rate (0–10) how much stress they experienced as a child and inquire about their reasons for the number chosen. The Hidden Stress Screening Test additionally includes two items from the Patient Health Questionnaire (PHQ-9), two items from the General Anxiety Disorder-7 (GAD-7), and two items from the PTSD Checklist for DSM-5 (PCL-5). These are screenings for DSM-5 criteria of major depression, generalized anxiety, and posttraumatic stress disorder, respectively. Assessing psychiatric history and current psychological functioning is important for understanding the patient's symptoms in context. Clarke and colleagues (2019) also suggest clinicians further listen for generalized statements of fatigue and emotional distress. Examples include "I cannot take this anymore," "I am just so exhausted and worn out," or "I've reached my limit."

Workability Assessment

Once the clinician has an understanding of the patient's life context, problem context, and stress context, they can start formulating a conceptualization of the patient's symptoms. Specifically, the clinician conceptualizes the patient's pain and pain management strategies within the patient's unique life and health context. This includes assessing the workability of the patient's current strategies, and connecting this back to the patient's values. Robinson's (2020) Contextual Assessment as well as the focusing questions used in FACT (Strosahl et al., 2012) can help structure this part of the evaluation.

1   Valued Direction: *What are you seeking? Who and what matters most to you? What direction would you like your life to take? What actions would you like to see yourself doing more, less, or differently that would tell you that you were moving in the "right" direction? What would you do if your pain was no longer a problem for you?* The clinician can also use some variation of the Miracle Question: *If a miracle occurred and you woke up tomorrow and your life was exactly how you would like it to be, what would that look like? What would you be doing? What kind of person would you be? How would you know that you were living your life in a meaningful way?* The purpose of these questions is to understand what the patient would do if they had reduced pain and/or greater function. The patient's answers highlight their values and often naturally translate into functional behavioral goals of treatment.

2   Current Strategies: *What have you tried? What pain management and coping strategies are you currently using? What strategies have you used in the past? What are the "rules" for your pain management?* Listen carefully for avoidance-based strategies. This is also an opportunity to reinforce the patient's problem-solving efforts, validate their distress, and learn from what has not worked.

3   Workability of Strategies: *How are these strategies working for you? Has your pain been reduced? What is or has been the cost of these strategies* (short-term and long-term)? *How are your relationships and activities impacted?*

This data helps the clinician understand not only the workability of the patient's strategies, but also the workability of their expectations or goals. Persistent pain or psychosomatic symptoms can lead to poor health outcomes as the result of chronically unfulfilled goals and rigid pursuit of unrealistic measures of success. Flexible goal adjustment may be necessary to establish goals that are both personally meaningful and achievable within the patient's life and health context.

Chakra Assessment

During the initial interview, the clinician is listening for where the patient is experiencing disconnection within their body, self, and values-based action. This requires identifying the patient's location and quality of somatic symptoms, painful emotional content, self-perceptions, and values. These are all clues as to which chakra(s) may be most in need of balancing and healing. There are several methods for determining which chakras(s) to target for initial intervention. Change anywhere in the system can have meaningful effects for the patient, but the goal of COACT is to select a pivot point where the slightest change is likely to have the greatest impact.

The simplest approach is to be guided by the patient's prominent somatic symptoms. The location of symptoms is interpreted as evidence of chakra dysfunction, and treatment can begin by targeting healing in the associated chakra. However, for more complex cases, clinicians may want to consider other aspects of the chakra system. Once the clinician is more familiar with the chakras, they will likely be able to identify patterns and areas of dysfunction rather easily. For learning and training purposes, the Brief Chakra Assessment (Appendix C) may be used to guide this process. For each key domain (body, self, values), the clinician circles or underlines the patient's symptom information in the chart to identify which chakra is primarily impacted: 1) Where does the patient primarily experience pain and/or discomfort in their body?; 2) What traits or self-perspectives have been lost due to control-based pain management strategies?; 3) What painful emotions are prominent?; 4) What values have been sacrificed in efforts to control pain? For example, a patient presents with recurring chest pain with no medical diagnosis. He shares feelings of resentment for painful experiences in his past, and has few close relationships. He is currently in the process of divorce, and has withdrawn from his usual friendships and activities. For this patient, intervention at the heart chakra may be the most impactful.

Selecting a chakra target can also be done more collaboratively. The Circle of Pain Awareness Worksheet (Appendix D) guides the patient through their own brief chakra assessment. Clinicians invite patients to write-in their physical pain symptoms, their painful emotions, their desired self-traits, and their values. The clinician highlights how the patient's strategies to avoid or control their pain (i.e., push these experiences outside the circle of awareness and disconnect from the body), also disconnects them from their self and values. The clinician and patient then discuss how the patient can accept pain into their awareness in order to also contact their true Self and values.

Clinicians may also seek to determine in which core domain (nonattachment, somatic awareness, self-integration, values-based action) the patient appears to have the least developed skills. The COACT Skills Assessment (Appendix E) summarizes specific behaviors associated with each skill to assist identification of strengths and weaknesses. Clinicians may then complete a partial chakra assessment to determine which chakra may be most imbalanced within a particular domain (body, self, values). The patient's report of somatic symptoms reflects chakra dysfunction in the body. To assess disconnection from self-perspectives or values, clinicians and patients can use the Self-Assessment Worksheet (Appendix F) or the Values Assessment Worksheet (Appendix G). Both worksheets provide examples of self-traits or values, respectively, that are associated with each chakra. The patient is asked to select a few self-traits or values that are most important to them, and then reflect on how their pain management strategies may interfere with the expression of these self-traits or values. The patient also indicates on a scale of 0 (never) to 4 (nearly always) how consistent their actions are with the selected traits or values. Only a few traits and values are provided on the worksheets. If a patient suggests a term that is not listed, the clinician should review Chapter 4 and use their best judgment to determine which chakra is most likely indicated. Areas for intervention may be based on the traits and values chosen as most important to the patient, or where the patient reports the greatest incongruence.

Lastly, clinicians may simply start intervention at the root chakra. For many patients, if not most, root chakra dysfunction will be a key component of their psychosomatic distress. This is because the root chakra contributes to one's sense of safety, stability, and trust, which are significantly impacted by experiences of stress and trauma. Grounding and restoring healthy energy in this chakra is important for calming the sympathetic nervous system, the body's stress response, and for establishing a sense of safety and security. The root chakra also serves as a foundation for the entire system, and improving health in the root chakra can similarly provide a foundation for treatment.

Creative Hopelessness

To be ready for change, patients will need to accept that their current strategies for coping with pain or somatic symptoms are 1) not really effective, and/or, 2) costly in terms of other aspects of their life that have been given up. This realization is an important step towards the patient being open to trying something different. ACT refers to this stage of treatment as fostering "creative hopelessness," meaning the patient realizes the hopelessness of their pain avoidant ("control-and-eliminate") strategies and begins to consider alternatives (Hayes et al., 2012). It is the patient's strategies, not the patient themselves, that is hopeless. Additionally, the patient's strategies may have previously been useful, but have become unworkable due to changing contexts. Strategies developed when coping with acute stress, such as ignoring the body or painful emotions, may have helped the patient tune-out pain in order to focus on their survival needs. However, these same strategies are now interfering with the patient pursuing their values and improving their health. ACT has a number of metaphors used to demonstrate the concept of creative hopelessness.

1   Man in the Hole: Imagine you are wandering through a field with just a small bag of tools. You have been told that these tools will prepare you for anything you might encounter. You are not sure where you are headed, but you are carefully moving onward. Suddenly you fall into a large hole. It is dark and you can hardly see the top of the hole. At first you feel quite defeated, and then you remember your tool bag. You are sure that something in there can help you get out of this predicament. You reach in the bag and discover that the only tool is a shovel. Seeing no other options, you start digging. After a while you stop and check your progress. You find that even with all your hard work, the hole has only gotten bigger! You try digging even faster, working until your arms feel weak. No matter how hard you try, the hole only gets bigger. Your small shovel eventually breaks. You sit there wishing you had a larger, indestructible shovel. Finally, you see the shadow of someone walking by near the top of the hole. You call out, and what do you ask for? A bigger shovel! Sometimes we get "tunnel vision," and can only see one way of doing things, no matter how much this way does not work. Where do you think you might be digging in your life? (Hayes et al., 2012).

2   Room of Adhesive Tape: Imagine your life is like a room. There is a storm that causes some damage to the ceiling, and now there is a small leak. You patch the leak with some adhesive tape, and instantly feel better. Then the water leaks through the tape, and you have to repair it again. This happens over and over again. Then other leaks start showing up. You move quickly to place tape over each one, and then repair as needed. Before you know it, you are spending more and more of your time trying to tape up these leaks, and more and more water is getting into the room.

3   Biofeedback/Polygraph: A popular misstep in the pursuit of symptom resolution is to focus too much on the goal. ACT uses the metaphor of being connected to biofeedback equipment or a polygraph machine while someone holds a gun to your head to demonstrate the paradox of control. You are told to relax, or they will pull the trigger. Can you relax? This may sound absurd and yet this is what many essentially do to themselves all the time! "I have to focus on this test or my life will be over!" "I need to get a good night's sleep or I will lose my job!" (Hayes et al., 2012).

Reframe the Problem

Once the clinician has enough information for a functional contextual understanding of the patient's symptom(s), the symptom is reframed for the patient according to this formulation. The process here is to normalize, validate, reframe, activate. Clinicians normalize the patient's pain and pain management efforts, validate their distress, reframe the problem as ineffective coping strategies (e.g., avoidance), and support the patient in taking action that will help them cope more effectively and move towards their values (Hayes, 2019). The purpose is to convey that the patient's pain or somatic symptom is not the problem, but rather their relationship to their pain and control efforts create conflict. Clinicians seek to support the client in questioning the accuracy and usefulness of their current strategies, which opens them to a reconceptualization of their distress (Strosahl et al., 2012). There are several ACT metaphors that can help illustrate the problem with avoidance.

1   Hungry Tiger: One day you find a sweet tiger cub meowing outside. She is adorable and playful, so you decide to bring her inside and keep her as a pet. She continues to meow and you guess she might be hungry. You feed her some raw beef from your freezer, and continue to feed her every day. She grows bigger and bigger, and needs more and more food. She no longer meows when hungry, but growls aggressively. The sweet little kitten is now a full-grown tiger that could make you its next meal if she got hungry enough. Your pain can be thought of like this tiger. Each time you avoid your pain, it's like feeding it a big piece of meat. This feeding helps your pain grow bigger and stronger. In the moment, this seems like the easiest and quickest way of dealing with it. However, over time, feeding your pain gives it more power and greater control over you (Hayes, 2019).

2   Pancakes: Do **not** think about pancakes. Do not do it! What comes to mind? You are probably thinking about exactly pancakes or something that is decidedly *not* pancakes. Either way, your next thoughts were determined by the idea of pancakes. Even to verify that your thought is *not* something, you still have to hold that content in your mind, which leads to ongoing reminders of the original or undesired content and a strengthened neural pathway of this response. This is why avoidant strategies do not work, and most of the time actually increase distressing content.

3   Hot Stove: Have you ever touched a hot stove or some other hot surface? If so, you likely experienced immediate pain that prompted you to move your hand away, right? Having your hand burned cued you to take quick action to prevent further damage. What would happen if you did not get burned? You might have left your hand on the stove and suffered great damage to your hand. While the burn was

painful, it actually saved you from far greater pain. Additionally, what would happen if you decided never to use the stove out of fear that you might get burned? You would be limited in your ability to feed yourself and your values of fulfilling your basic needs would be secondary to your desire for pain avoidance (Hayes, 2019).

Making the Mind-Body Connection

Clinicians provide education on the mind-body connection, and guide patients to understand their pain in the context of their own life and stress. Some patients may have already been suspecting a psychological factor was involved in causing or exacerbating their symptoms, while others will need more education and support to understand how the mind and body are each contributing to their symptoms (Clarke et al., 2019). The clinician may explain how thoughts, feelings, and memories all influence how the body functions, and how the mind makes interpretations and decisions based on sensations and messages from the body. It is important to communicate that the mind-body relationship is bidirectional, and that both components play an equal role in one's health. In suggesting that the patient's pain or somatic symptoms are related to psychological processes, the clinician is not claiming the distress is invalid, not "real", or "all in their head." If a patient makes this misinterpretation, the clinician should provide validation and reassure the patient that their pain is being taken seriously. The clinician can provide further education on how stress and lifestyle factors influence different systems in the body. For example, the clinician may explain how stress alters different functions in the sympathetic nervous system. Similarly, the clinician can explain how the mind often looks to the body for help in determining feelings. When the heart is beating faster than usual, for example, the mind takes that as a clue and looks for other signs that might help explain the cause of this sensation. Depending on what other clues or messages are available, the mind may conclude the individual is excited or anxious. Clinicians explain that treatment will include interventions for both the mind and the body, and focus on restoring healthy communication between the two.

Sharing the Conceptualization

Clinicians offer a conceptualization of the patient's symptom, highlighting current rules of pain avoidance and the mind-body connection. This conceptualization includes a summary of the patient's physical symptoms, self-perceptions, emotional distress, and values related to their pain experience. The conceptualization draws upon chakra theory, but the clinician can choose to specify this part of the model or not. Some patients may be interested in a brief explanation regarding how different energy centers in the body are associated with specific physical and psychological experiences. Others may have a negative response to terms like "yoga," "chakras," or "energy." In most cases, a general statement would be acceptable. For example, "Our mind and body influence each other in many ways. Certain thoughts or feelings can actually contribute to physical sensations, and vice versa. It is not always clear how these relationships work, but there are some common connections." The clinician then moves towards their conceptualization of the patient's specific symptom presentation. "You and I have been looking at a number of issues and concerns that you have in regards to your pain. However, some themes seem to be appearing. This is how I see it, and I would certainly be interested in your thoughts. It seems to me that in trying to manage your nausea and stomach pain, you have felt powerless and frustrated. You have had to give up several of your usual activities, which you feel has lowered your self-confidence and self-esteem. Am I getting that right?" This phrasing invites immediate feedback from the client, and invites them to collaborate with the clinician in conceptualizing their symptom and guiding treatment. Another example, "It seems to me that your knee pain is causing you a great deal of distress. I hear that this pain makes you feel anxious and worried about your ability to get around and take care of yourself. It makes sense to me that you try to ignore this pain as much as possible, and distract yourself from your anxiety. I also understand that you stopped playing tennis because of the pain, and that this has been difficult for you because you really enjoy being physically active. It seems like in trying to get rid of your pain and worry, you have also had to give up something important to you." In this example, the clinician's response normalizes and validates the patient's response, emphasizes the avoidance or activity given up, and connects this with the patient's values.

Fostering Nonattachment

Once the clinician and patient have agreed on a definition of the problem and direction for treatment, the first step is to begin developing a stance of nonattachment. To let go of attachments using the psychological flexibility model, clinicians emphasize acceptance and defusion skills. Separating from attachments allows the patient to start changing the context and function of their pain symptoms. Below are some examples of pain-related attachments associated with each chakra.

1   Root: family/cultural beliefs about pain (e.g. fight through the pain, do not talk about painful emotions, self-care is selfish), hypervigilance to pain, health anxiety, fears about ongoing pain
2   Sacral: limiting fun/enjoyable activities to avoid pain, desire for control, excessive pleasure-seeking, blaming oneself for their pain, viewing experience of pain as a punishment

3   Solar Plexus: competitive attitude towards pain ("I can beat this!"), believing experience of pain indicates a weakness, feeling powerless to experience of pain, anger towards or about pain

4   Heart: rigid beliefs about pain experience being "unfair," self-sacrificial behaviors and taking care of other's needs instead of their own, beliefs that one is entitled to special treatment because of their pain/treating others poorly because of their pain

5   Throat: beliefs that one has little to offer or contribute because of their pain, poor/excessive communication about their pain, viewing their pain or related behaviors from a morality perspective, judging oneself or comparing pain experience to others' (e.g. "I should not feel this way when others have it way worse")

6   Brow: limited perspective about pain, conceptualized pain narratives, unable to imagine other possibilities or life without pain, engaging in behaviors that increase pain with little awareness or insight

Defusion and acceptance skills help the patient begin to make room for their pain and their experience, and to separate from their mental rules of pain avoidance. To quickly demonstrate the effects of acceptance and defusion, ask the patient to place their hand out in front of them. Have the patient hold their palm just in front of their face, and imagine their hand represents their pain. Notice how this interferes with their ability to see clearly. What would it be like to go through life like this? This physical metaphor demonstrates how cognitive fusion consumes one's awareness. Then ask the patient to completely extend their arm, still with their hand in front of their face, but now much farther out. Notice any difficulty or discomfort with holding the arm out like this. What would it be like to go through life like this? This demonstrates the struggle of avoidance and pushing painful experiences away. Ask the patient to place their hand gently at their side. Notice how much easier it is to see and move through the world. The hand is still nearby, but no longer intruding on the patient's experience (Hayes, 2019). Defusion and acceptance skills help individuals find this balance of disentangling from their pain, while still carrying it near and making room for their pain in order to engage with life and their values.

Mindfulness

Mindfulness has two primary components in practice: 1) self-regulation of attention, and 2) orientation toward the present moment characterized by curiosity, openness, and acceptance (Hofmann et al., 2010). While mindfulness exercises tend to produce relaxation, the goal of mindfulness is to bring one's awareness into the moment and accept one's experience as it is. Stressors often draw attention elsewhere and contribute to negative thoughts and emotions. For example, excessive focus on the past often leads to depression while excessive focus on the future may cause anxiety

(Hofmann et al., 2010). Mindfulness-based treatments help individuals learn how to respond to stress "reflectively rather than reflexively" (Hofmann et al., 2010), and reduce repetitive negative thinking (Gu et al., 2015). Mindfulness thus enhances the flexibility skills of acceptance, defusion, and present moment attention. Mindfulness practices can be contextualized to promote somatic awareness (described in the following chapter), as well as engage chakra energy. Some ways to focus mindfulness practice for each chakra are: 1) Root: smell, physical activity (e.g. walking); 2) Sacral: taste, play activity; 3) Solar Plexus: sight, external images; 4) Heart: touch, breath; 5) Throat: sound/music, words; 6) Brow: mental imagery, colors.

General Acceptance Interventions

The primary process of change in ACT for chronic pain is pain acceptance. Only when one allows their complete experience into their awareness, unchanged and authentic, can they honestly pursue their values. Pain acceptance does not mean they must *like* being in pain, but that they can tolerate the reality of their pain and choose not to fight against this experience. Several metaphors used in the ACT literature highlight the importance of acceptance and willingness to hold one's experiences with integrity.

1   Quicksand: Have you ever heard of quicksand? As quicksand causes people to sink, the immediate instinct is to fight against this and try to push oneself out. However, this is exactly what makes the problem worse. The more you struggle, the deeper you sink. The best way to survive is to lay down and spread as much of your body weight across the surface as you can. To give up the fight may seem counterintuitive, but embracing the quicksand in this way is what allows you to get unstuck. The same is true with pain and distress. Accepting the pain is what gives us the best chance for surviving and getting through it (Hayes, 2019).

2   Unwelcome Party Guest: Imagine you are having a house party. You have invited all your neighbors, family, and friends. Guests start arriving and you are very excited. Then your heart sinks as someone you deliberately did not invite walks in. He is obnoxious, rude, and tends to demand a lot. However, you do not want to disrupt the party or hurt anyone's feelings. Can you welcome him into your home while also being disappointed that he is here? You do not have to like him to offer him some food and a drink. Or you can decide to throw him out, but then what else might happen? He might cause further disruption on his way out. If he came with someone you invited, that person might be upset. What if he keeps trying to find his way back in? Do you really want to spend your party guarding the front door? Ultimately it is your choice how you respond. What action allows you to have the best time at your party? (*Joe the Bum*, Hayes et al., 2012).

3   Emperor Moth: Imagine you find an emperor moth cocoon outside. Excitedly, you go and check on it once, maybe even several times each day. You hope to witness the moth emerging from the cocoon. One day you go out and see that the moth is just starting to appear. You watch it struggle to push its way out, making slow progress. Then a few minutes go by and nothing seems to be happening. Worried, you decide to help. You get some small scissors and open the cocoon so that the moth easily gets out. You wait for the moth to spread its wings and fly off, but it does not. Instead, its wings are shriveled up and it cannot fly. The moth needed to experience pushing its way out of the cocoon in order to strengthen its body and wings. It could only fly after this painful struggle. Without this struggle, it could never be a healthy moth.

Contextualized Acceptance Interventions (*Pain and Chakra-Based*)

These interventions are specific for pain acceptance, and can be further contextualized to chakra-specific experiences of physical or emotional pain (fear, guilt/blame, anger/shame, jealousy/resentment and grief, judgment/doubt, depression/despair).

1   A Caring Exercise (Hayes, 2019, p. 203–204). Choose an experience you have difficulty accepting (i.e. your pain) and use a metaphor for holding it gently. The metaphor can further be contextualized to use themes and imagery associated with a particular chakra.

(I)   Root: Inhale your experience (take it in) like the smell of a flower or fresh grass. "Hold your experience like a delicate flower in your hand"

(II)   Sacral: Savor your experience like a bite of your favorite dessert. "Take in your experience like a drink of pure water"

(III)   Solar plexus: Observe your experience like the flickering flames of a birthday candle. Witness your experiences like a roaring bonfire.

(IV)   Heart: Hold your experience like a soft pillow. "Embrace your experience like a crying child." "Inhale your experience like a deep breath"

(V)   Throat: Sing to your experience like it is a sleeping child. Listen to your experience like you would a dear friend.

(VI)   Brow: Look at your experience like an artistic masterpiece. Internalize your experience like the wisdom of a master.

2   Mindfulness: Mindfulness practice engages many psychological flexibility skills. It is discussed in further detail in Chapter 7 as a tool for developing flexible attention to the moment and somatic awareness. However, mindfulness is also a practice of non-judgmental acceptance, and can be further contextualized to the different chakras.

(I) Root: mindful physical activity
(II) Sacral: mindful play
(III) Solar Plexus: mindful eating
(IV) Heart: mindful breathing
(V) Throat: mindful words
(VI) Brow: mindful imagery

3   Carry it with you (Hayes, 2019): Invite the patient to write down a painful thought, feeling, sensation, etc., and carry this piece of paper with them. The patient does this to bring their pain "along for the ride," while continuing to perform their usual activities.

4   Accepting Posture: Patients can practice adopting an open and accepting attitude towards their unwanted private events by visualizing themselves as something flexible and fluid. The imagery used can be contextualized to a specific chakra. Patients may practice responding like a bendy tree (root), ocean wave (sacral), dancing flame (solar plexus), gust of wind (heart), musical note or reverberating sound (throat), or bouncing light (third-eye).

General Defusion Interventions

In order to make room for pain, individuals also need to confront the rules of pain avoidance they have been using for symptom management. These rules were designed to push pain out of their experience, although likely unsuccessfully. These rules have to be challenged and released, therefore, in order to hold one's pain honestly. General metaphors and exercises can again be used to introduce the idea of defusion and move the patient towards greater flexibility of thought.

1   Zoom In/Zoom Out: Sometimes we get so absorbed into something we are watching or looking at, that we actually feel part of the events. Have you ever been to an IMAX theater? These large screens help us feel part of the action. Even in a regular movie theater, we might get so pulled in that we forget, even for a moment, that we are watching a film. Our minds can do this to us too. The mind feeds us thoughts, images, feelings, or memories and magnifies them. We are looking at the contents of our mind up close, and get absorbed into their stories. What helps us defuse is to zoom out rather than zooming in. Rather than being immersed in the story like when watching a movie, we take a step back to observe our mind from a detached distance.

2   Repetition: Repetition is a standard defusion technique that originated with Edward Titchener. It typically takes about thirty seconds for individuals to defuse the sound and meaning of the word, such that the vocalization of the word is most prominent in their awareness. As the individual's attention is pulled to ward the sound of the

word, the meaning holds less weight (Hayes, 2019). Repetition is best used by condensing a particular thought to the shortest meaningful unit. Using longer or more complete sentences makes it more difficult to defuse sound and meaning. For example, the thought "I have to focus on other people or my pain will take over my life" might become "take over."

3   Reprogramming Pain: Chronic pain is a learned response in the central nervous system. First, clinicians can demonstrate how easily the brain can be programmed to generate automatic responses. Ask the patient to finish these sentences: Mary had a little _____. Twinkle, twinkle, little _____. Humpty Dumpty sat on a _____. How did the patient know what word goes in each blank? The brain was programmed to know these rhymes through many repetitions. Similarly, through repeated experiences of pain, the brain has learned to generate a chronic pain response. How likely is it that an individual could unlearn the lyrics to classic nursery rhyme? Extremely unlikely! However, could they learn new songs that reduce the importance of this rhyme? Absolutely! As people learn new associations and have different experiences, old programming becomes less and less important. Whatever is repeated and rehearsed will become the prominent program.

Contextualized Defusion Interventions (Pain and Chakra-Based)

1   Leaves on a Stream: A common ACT defusion technique is to observe one's thoughts as leaves floating down a stream (Hayes et al., 2012). The individual is instructed to imagine placing each thought on a leaf as it floats by to encourage passive observation and letting the thought go. This exercise can be contextualized with chakra-based imagery and themes.

> (I)   Root: leaves falling off a tree, petals off a flower
> (II) Sacral: waves crashing on the beach, raindrops falling
> (III) Solar Plexus: ash or smoke floating out of fire
> (IV) Heart: clouds in the sky, wind blowing away dandelions
> (V)   Throat: musical notes, soldiers on parade holding each thought/ feeling on a poster
> (VI) Third Eye: light across a rainbow, lightning bolts striking

2   Defuse with Exercise (Root): Individuals can engage the body in physical activity in order to reduce the intensity of distressing thoughts or feelings. Engaging in exercise and physical activity has long been used to improve one's mood and overall health. Regular exercise is often recommended for stress management, and is used in Dialectical Behavior Therapy (DBT; Linehan, 2014) for coping with overwhelming emotions.

3   Laughter is the Best Medicine (Sacral): Laughter helps relax the mind and body, and is great for defusion. During experiences of extreme

stress, it can be difficult to find humor. When people are hurting, their experience tends to feel very dark and heavy. Humor and playfulness bring light. Most people have a few memories or experiences from their life that make them laugh just thinking about it. Invite patients to share some of these funny moments. Patients may come up with a key word or phrase that serves as a reminder of this memory, and then use this to help pull up this memory when they need a little laughter.

4   Powerful Disobedience (Solar Plexus): Personal and willpower can be used to promote defusion by emphasizing the limitations of the mind and language: we can say one thing and do another (Hayes, 2019). For example, the individual can walk around while saying, "I cannot walk around" or make a fist while saying "I cannot make a fist." Individuals can also write or make false statements about their opinions (e.g. "I hate ice cream") to further demonstrate how thoughts are not always factual.

5   Defusing Breath (Heart): Focusing attention in the present or on a fixed point can help release mental attachments. Rather than getting hooked by painful thoughts, feelings, or sensations, individuals can maintain a neutral, detached stance by bringing awareness to their breath. Individuals may find it helpful to think "here" on each inhale and "now" on each exhale.

6   Singing/Silly Voices (Throat): Techniques that disrupt the intensity or literality of a mental event are excellent for quick defusion. ACT clinicians often use exercises that undermine the seriousness or pain associated with a particular thought by saying the thought in a silly voice or singing it (Hayes et al., 2012). Individuals can form the thought into a sentence and then sing it in their head or out loud to a familiar tune (e.g., "Happy Birthday, "Row, Row, Row Your Boat"). They can also experiment with different paces (slowed down or sped up) and voices (e.g. cartoon voice, celebrity voice, higher/lower, accents, etc.). This exercise is not designed for the patient to ridicule themselves, but simply to make room for a different way of relating to the painful event.

7   Externalizing Pain (Brow): There are a number of techniques that can be used to externalize and/or personify one's pain experience in order to promote defusion (Hayes et al., 2012; Strosahl et al., 2012).

   (I) Name It: Using language that distinguishes oneself from their pain helps defuse one's self-concept from their experience of pain. Individuals may say, "My mind/body/pain says…" to clearly distinguish between these experiences and themselves. Patients can even give their pain experience a name and then respond with something like, "Charlie is really making it difficult for me to get my work done today."

   (II) Describe It: One can externalize their pain experience by describing it in physicalizing and non-evaluative terms. What does it look like? Describe the color, texture, size, and form of the pain. (*Physicalizing*, Hayes et al., 2012).

(III) Thank It: By defusing from their pain, patients have the choice to listen to their pain, appreciate what their pain (also body or mind) is trying to tell them, and make a decision that moves them in the direction of their values. In most cases of chronic pain, the mind and body's alarm systems are malfunctioning, and messages of pain are not reliable indications of any threat or danger. An example response might be, "Thank you, pain/mind/body for trying to keep me safe, but I'm okay" or "I appreciate your trying to help, but I can handle this."

References

Clarke, D. D. (n.d.). Hidden stress screening test. Retrieved on February 7, 2022, from https://ppdassociation.org/resources/#stress-test.

Clarke, D. D., Schubiner, H., Clark-Smith, M., & Abbass, A. (Eds) (2019). *Psychophysiologic Disorders: Trauma Informed, Interprofessional Diagnosis and Treatment*. Psychophysiologic Disorders Association.

Felitti, V. J., Anda, R. F., Nordenberg, D., Williamson, D. F., Spitz, A. M., Edwards, V., Koss, M. P., & Marks, J. S. (1998) Relationship of childhood abuse and household dysfunction to many of the leading causes of death in adults. The adverse childhood experiences (ACE) study. *American Journal of Preventive Medicine*, 14(4), 245–258.

Gu, J., Strauss, C., Bond, R., & Cavanagh, K. (2015). How do mindfulness-based cognitive therapy and mindfulness-based stress reduction improve mental health and wellbeing? A systematic review and meta-analysis of mediation studies. *Clinical Psychology Review*, 37, 1–12.

Hayes, S. C. (2019). *A liberated mind: How to pivot toward what matters*. Avery.

Hayes, S. C., Strosahl, K. D. & Wilson, K. G. (2012). *Acceptance and commitment therapy: The process and practice of mindful change* (2nd ed.). Guilford.

Hofmann, S. G., Sawyer, A. T., Witt, A. A., & Oh, D. (2010). The effect of mindfulness-based therapy on anxiety and depression: A meta-analytic review. *Journal of Consulting and Clinical Psychology*, 78(2), 169–183.

Hooper, L. M., Stockton, P., Krupnick, J., & Green, B. L. (2011). The development, use, and psychometric properties of the trauma history questionnaire. *Journal of Loss and Trauma*, 16, 258–283.

Kroenke K, Spitzer R. L., & Williams, J. B. (2002). The PHQ-15: Validity of a new measure for evaluating the severity of somatic symptoms. *Psychosomatic Medicine*, 64(2), 258–266,

Linehan, M. M. (2014). *DBT Skills Training Manual*, 2nd Edition. Guilford Press.

Robinson, P. J., (2020). *Basics of behavior change in primary care*. Springer.

Strosahl, K., Robinson, P., & Gustavsson, T. (2012). *Brief interventions for radical change: Principles & practice of focused acceptance & commitment therapy*. New Harbinger.

Weathers, F. W., Blake, D. D., Schnurr, P. P., Kaloupek, D. G., Marx, B. P., & Keane, T. M. (2013). The Life Events Checklist for DSM-5 (LEC-5) – Standard [Measurement instrument].

7 Somatic Awareness

Somatic Awareness

Tantra and many yoga practices emphasize using the body as a tool for self-actualization. This chapter describes several interventions and exercises used to promote somatic awareness and mind-body communication through mindfulness and relaxation techniques. It is recommended that patients be presented with a wide variety of options so that they can determine which exercises are the best fit for them. Patients are encouraged to practice these techniques during clinical visits and at home.

Somatic awareness reflects the ability to notice subtle changes within the body in response to both external and internal climates. Greater somatic awareness can be helpful or harmful depending on one's attentional biases, or orientation towards their physiologic sensations (Ginzburg et al, 2015). When associated with catastrophizing attributions of body sensations, somatic awareness increases attentional focus on pain, pain perception, anxiety, and body distress. However, when associated with non-judgmental acceptance (i.e. mindfulness) of body sensations, somatic awareness can attenuate the experience of pain and enhance pain habituation, which may be reduced or absent in the patients with chronic pain (Defrin et al., 2015). The development of somatic awareness in itself, therefore, is not as important in the treatment of psychosomatic conditions as is developing flexible and mindful attention to the body's sensations.

There are six major approaches to relaxation used by health professionals: yoga stretching, breathing exercises, progressive muscle relaxation, autogenic training, imagery, and meditation. These methods are generally found to be interchangeable and equally useful, prompting most therapists to rely primarily on one or two preferred relaxation techniques (Ghoncheh & Smith, 2004). Clinicians providing Chakra-Organized ACT (COACT) may integrate their own preferred methods; however, this chapter will present mindfulness, muscle relaxation, yoga postures, and breathing techniques. All of these interventions help develop flexible attention to the body's sensations and generally promote relaxation through activation of the parasympathetic nervous system, the counterpart to the sympathetic nervous system or

DOI: 10.4324/9781003251293-8

Table 7.1 Chakras and Body Areas

Root	*Sacral*	*Solar Plexus*	*Heart*	*Throat*	*Brow*
lower back, legs, feet	genito-pelvic area, hips	abdomen, middle spine	chest, upper back, shoulders, arms	mouth, neck	head, eyes, ears, nose

"fight-or-flight" response. These skills also develop interoception (awareness within the body) and proprioception (awareness of the body in space). The Somatic Awareness Tracking worksheet (see Appendix H) can be used to record when one practices somatic awareness their observations of the experience. Each skill can further be tailored to focus on body areas associated with a particular chakra (see Table 7.1).

Cautionary Notes

It is important to gather a detailed medical history to avoid recommending somatic interventions that may negatively impact pre-existing medical conditions. Patients should be informed of the potential risks and benefits of all exercises. Regarding yoga postures particularly, the clinician should be honest about their level of training (if any) and competency using yoga stretches with therapy. Patients may be referred to a trained yoga instructor if they are interested in a more in-depth yoga practice. Joanna Spence, author of *Trauma-Informed Yoga: A Toolbox for Therapists* (2021), recommends searching for yoga classes with "gentle" or "restorative" in the title, and classes that emphasize breathing techniques.

Additionally, engaging with the body can be uncomfortable or even triggering for those with prior trauma experiences. It is important that clinicians provide clear directions and expectations before beginning a somatic exercise technique. Clinicians should use open and invitational language, create a safe and welcoming space, establish clear boundaries, normalize symptoms or responses to movement that may arise for patients, and avoid any physical touch without the patient's clear consent (Spence, 2021). Clinicians should also check-in with the patient before, during, and after the somatic exercise. Patients should not be pushed to engage in any somatic exercise they do not feel comfortable with.

Mindfulness

Mindfulness may be the most widely used mind-body intervention. Jon Kabat-Zinn, the creator of mindfulness-based stress reduction (MBSR), led the empirical study of mindfulness in psychotherapy science. He defined mindfulness from its use in Western Buddhism as intentional attention to the present moment without judgment. Kabat-Zinn studied mindfulness as a practice and therapeutic technique, and developed MBSR originally for the treatment of chronic pain. MBSR is an empirically supported treatment that primarily teaches three mindfulness-based exercises: body scan, sitting meditation, and gentle yoga. Mindfulness-based treatments improve physical and psychological wellbeing through improved attentional control, experiential acceptance, empathy, stress reduction, and interoception (Hofmann et al., 2010). Mindfulness is also associated with reductions in pain intensity, and increases in pain threshold and tolerance (Zeidan et al., 2011).

There are many ways to focus flexible attention through mindfulness in order to develop somatic awareness and engage the chakras. Attention may be directed towards body sensations, sensory experiences, mental images, words, and other internal or external material. The content selected for concentration can facilitate engagement of a particular chakra. The chosen concentration point acts like a "home base" for the individual to focus and refocus their attention when they notice their mind wandering or objectivity being lost. Regardless of what focal point is used, the functional process remains the same: holding attention on a fixed point while practicing nonattachment. As discussed in the previous chapter, a stance of nonattachment involves observation, acceptance, and defusion.

Mindfulness Exercises

1 Sitting Meditation: While sitting in a comfortable position, bring your awareness into your body. Observe what is going on both around you and within you. The goal is to bring your presence completely into the moment. Your mind and attention will naturally wander. This is an opportunity to practice defusion and acceptance techniques. Allow your thoughts to pass through your mind, and gently bring your attention back to the present.

2 Sensory Meditations: Mindful meditation often encourages sensory awareness. Gradually focus attention on each of your senses, or focus on one sensory experience to engage a particular chakra (Root-smell; Sacral-taste; Solar Plexus-sight; Heart-touch; Throat-sound and vibration; Brow-light and intuition).

3 Body Scan: Lie comfortably on your back with your hands at your sides, palms up. Take deep, full breaths, and track the path of your breath through your body. Follow your inhale through your nose down into your diaphragm and stomach, and then follow the exhale back up. The goal of the body scan is to bring awareness to sensations throughout the body. Gradually begin with bringing awareness to your toes. Wiggle your toes and pay attention to the sensations. Take a breath and move your awareness to your feet and ankles. As you move through your body, observe if you experience any tightness or soreness. When you do, take a breath, and practice releasing that attachment with defusion, and acceptance. Next bring awareness to your shins, knees, and thighs. Bring your attention fully into each

body part for at least one to two full breaths. Hold your attention next on your pelvis, then stomach. What can you notice? Move your attention into your chest and heart. Can you hear or feel your heartbeat? Next is your throat and mouth. What does your breath feel like here? Finally notice each of your senses, your face, and the top of your head. Take several breaths and feel your entire body being supported by the ground beneath you. When you are ready, gently sit up and assess if you notice any changes in how your body feels.

4 Mindful Physical Activity (Root): Mindfulness can be practiced while walking, jogging, or otherwise engaging the physical body. It is important to wear comfortable clothes and shoes that will not be restricting or distracting. While walking, bring your awareness to each small movement. Notice how it feels to put one foot forwards, place your heel on the ground, and shift your weight to the toes as the other foot comes forward. Bring awareness to how the ground feels beneath your feet. Does the body feel strong and flexible or do movements feel uncoordinated and restricted? Is there any pain? How does the movement relax, energize, or tire the body?

5 Mindful Play (Sacral): Practice mindful awareness while engaging in an activity that is fun or pleasurable. Notice how the body responds to this activity, as well as any thoughts or feelings that show up. Do you notice any tension or relaxation in the body? What emotions are present?

6 Mindful Eating (Solar Plexus): Practicing mindfulness while eating is a popular technique. It involves noticing how it feels to bring the food to your mouth, taste and chew the food, and then swallow and hold the food in your stomach. Observe how your body responds to the food, does it feel nourished and energized? Does the body feel lethargic or slower after eating? Mindfulness can be used to check-in with one's hunger levels and listen to the body's cues regarding what foods to eat and how much.

7 Mindful Breathing (Heart): Practice taking diaphragmatic breaths and allow your awareness to follow the entirety of the breath cycle. Follow your breath through the nostrils, down through the throat into the lungs, diaphragm, and lower belly. Then notice the exhale in reverse.

8 Mindful Words (Throat): Practice mindful attention to words, either your words or other's words, and notice how these words influence sensations in the body. How does it feel in your body to say particular words or phrases? Think of statements you often make, and notice where the statement interacts with the body. Do these words produce pain, pleasure, relaxation, or other sensations? Bring mindful attention to the sensation of speaking, and observe how it feels to move your lips and tongue to produce sounds.

9   Mindful Music (Throat and Brow): Many people listen to music during mindful meditation. Notice how your body responds to the music. What sensations are present? Bring your awareness to the process of hearing, and what it feels like to listen closely to each note. Does the body relax? Are there notes or rhythms that produce tension?

10   Mindful Imagery (Brow): Mental imagery engages all the senses to create an internal experience. Practice bringing your full attention to a visualization or imagery exercise. You might follow a guided recording (many can be found online) or create your own visualization.

Muscle Relaxation

People naturally respond to pain and distress by tensing the body, which can exacerbate somatic symptoms. Each individual holds stress differently in the body, but muscle tension in the forehead, abdomen, neck, and shoulders are especially common. This tension produces a posture that is stiff and lacking in flexibility. If a person is habitually stressed, this posture and attitude also becomes a habit. Interventions that relax these muscles and loosen physical tension help produce mental relaxation and pain relief (Rama et al., 1976).

In yoga, systematic relaxation of the muscles is a tool for producing a calmer mental state. Most muscle relaxation interventions start with bringing one's attention to their toes or feet and slowly moving focus up through the body, concentrating on each sequential muscle group to promote a calm and relaxed state (Rama et al., 1976). Progressive muscle relaxation was first introduced in Western medicine by Edmund Jacobson in 1935 as a long procedure involving the tensing and relaxing of sixteen muscle groups. In 1948, Joseph Wolpe proposed abbreviated progressive muscle relaxation to focus on several muscle groups simultaneously, and many adaptations have been used since then. In its essence, progressive muscle relaxation involves training the body to voluntarily tense and then relax individual muscles from head to feet while the mind focuses on the contrasting sensations. Individuals may also focus muscle relaxation on parts of the body where they notice greater tension or somatic distress, or body areas associated with a particular chakra. This technique produces physiological and psychological relaxation by decreasing the individual's stress response, skeletal muscle contractions, and sensations of pain (Field, 2009). There is substantial empirical support for the use of progressive muscle relaxation with diverse symptom presentation, including anxiety, tension headaches, insomnia, chronic pain, inflammatory arthritis, and irritable bowel syndrome (McCallie et al., 2006). A cognitive-behavioral model offers several hypothesized mechanisms of action for progressive muscle relaxation, including tension relief (somatic and cognitive arousal reduction), disengagement from unnecessary goal-directed and analytic activity, and maintaining focus on simple stimuli (Smith et al., 1996).

Yoga Postures

Yoga has been labeled "embodied mindfulness" or "mindfulness in motion", as yoga movement engages many of the same mechanisms as mindfulness (Salmon et al., 2009). Most Westernized yoga practices emphasize three components: physical postures (asanas), breathing techniques (pranayama), and meditation (dyana). Yoga postures build a sense of agency and choice within body movements, which helps one feel a sense of control and rebuild trust with their body (Spence, 2021). Each posture engages specific body parts for different purposes.

From a yoga perspective, one's posture is both their physical and mental stance for interacting with the world (Rama et al., 1976). Physical form mirrors the mental state, and altering the body's posture can modify or enhance mental and emotional activity. When there is tension in part of the body, neighboring muscles often have to re-calibrate and adjust in an attempt to maintain the body's central balance. As the individual's physical and mental posture contributes to the misuse and weakening of certain muscles, it becomes more difficult to correct one's posture. Once aware of this misalignment, one has to slowly build back muscle strength. Many people spend most of the day in collapsed and slouched positions, often unconsciously, while watching television, working on a computer, or texting on their phones. These "culturally conditioned" positions have been found to enhance recall for negative and hopeless memories and reduce energy (Peper & Lin, 2012).

Benefits of Yoga Stretching

Through yoga, individuals learn to view themselves, their body, and the world differently. Yoga produces positive psychological benefits through increased self and body awareness, which leads to re-evaluation of one's self and values, increased tolerance and acceptance of the self, and engagement in other healthy activities (Anderzén-Carlsson et al., 2014).

Yoga improves health partially through moderation of the body's stress response. Greater frequency of yoga practice has been linked to better mental and physical health outcomes, including increased positive attitudes, vitality, relaxation, and anti-inflammatory hormones (Kiecolt-Glaser, et al., 2010). In diverse chronic pain patients, yoga interventions have produced improvements in quality of life and self-efficacy of chronic pain management, as well as reduced pain, pain interference in daily life, and physical disability (Büssing et al., 2012; Chang et al., 2016). Yoga interventions have also been used in populations with posttraumatic stress disorder (PTSD) to increase awareness of fear-related sensations in the body and counter avoidance symptoms (Emerson et al., 2009). Medical yoga shows similar health benefits and is intentionally designed for those with health conditions that would make it difficult for them to participate in a typical yoga class. The starting positions can be sitting, lying, or standing, and movements are slower (Anderzén-Carlsson et al., 2014).

Principles of Yoga Stretching

Yoga posture and body alignment should be flexible and contextually guided by the moment. Everyone's body is different. The goal is not to force the body into the "perfect" pose, which can cause pain and/or injury, but rather to balance stability, strength, and flexibility (Gordon et al., 2019). When the posture is fully controlled and stable, one experiences a natural ease and relaxed comfort. While practicing yoga poses, it is important to bring one's attention to the parts of the body engaged with the pose. This "tuning-in" and introspection helps to uncover and bring awareness to the sensations and feelings that may arise with each pose (Rama et al., 1976). This concentration also allows the individual to stay tuned-in with their body so as not to over-stretch, and potentially cause physical harm. If the posture is uncomfortable or painful, adjust or stop the pose. Once settled into a pose, individuals are encouraged to bring their attention to their breath, concentrating on smooth and steady breathing, and then bring their attention back to their body. While the pose relaxes the body in stillness, the breath keeps the body fluid and flexible (Rama et al., 1976). Some guiding principles to keep in mind:

1   Move only in a range of motion that does not increase pain.
2   Less is more. One can receive the benefits of yoga stretches without forcing the body into a deeper or more strenuous pose.
3   Go slow. Experiment with gentle movements and give the body time to adjust. Life often pushes people to pick up the pace and move quickly. Give yourself permission to slow down.
4   Watch your breath. Your breath should remain flexible and fluid. If you notice you are holding your breath or struggling to maintain a smooth rhythm, relax the pose.

Posture Support/Modifications

Yoga poses can, and should, be modified as needed for each individual. Most of the poses in this text can be done seated or standing. Common modifications include using pillows or folded blankets/towels for additional support. This extra cushion can be placed under joints or parts of the body to help promote ease of movement and comfort. Placing a pillow under the knees during Savasana, for example, can be helpful for those with back pain. Others may benefit from sitting on a folded-up blanket to slightly elevate their hips when sitting in a cross-legged posture. Yoga blocks, chairs, and walls can also be used for propping up and support, such as during bended poses. Straps are also commonly used when an individual cannot reach the body part they are extending towards (Gordon et al., 2019). Each individual is urged to listen to their own body when practicing any form of yoga or somatic exercise. Building this somatic awareness, after all, is the primary purpose of these exercises.

Yoga Postures for the Chakras

It is common for modern yoga practices to mention chakras and use different poses to engage a particular chakra. The techniques presented in this text are intentionally beginner's poses and simple exercises that can be taught and practiced even by those with no prior yoga experience. For each chakra, poses are presented in order from easiest to most advanced. Individuals are also encouraged to speak with local yoga instructors for more information and to ensure health and safety while practicing. Clinicians and patients should select poses according to the patient's chakra needs, while also being mindful of the patient's physical limits and medical comorbidities. Consultation with a medical professional and yoga instructor is strongly encouraged to rule out any contraindications for certain poses. The goal is not to try every pose or rush through several poses in a routine. Instead, clinicians should help the patient identify a few poses that work well for them, and encourage them to practice them with conscious intention. For treating psychosomatic symptoms and within the context of COACT, the goal of these yoga postures is to help promote somatic awareness and mental and physical relaxation. Practicing one to three poses regularly can help a patient learn how to build awareness within their body and chakra system. Each pose may be practiced or held for several minutes as the patient focuses on their breath to enhance body awareness.

Root Chakra: Grounding and Balancing

1 Mountain: Stand or sit upright with your feet hip-width apart. If standing, gently bend the knees to prevent locking. Ground through your feet by sinking your weight downward, pushing your energy towards the earth. Pull your shoulder blades slightly back, opening the chest. Keeping your gaze straight ahead, arms at your sides with palms facing forward and hands engaged with fingers pointed down. Breathe.

2 Tree: Stand with your feet parallel and touching so that your knees also meet. On an exhale, shift your weight onto your right foot, while bending your right knee slightly. Keep your spine straight and look forward while you gently lift your left foot off the ground. You can rest your toes on the ground and prop your foot up against your ankle. The bottom of your left foot is flat against the side of your right leg, toes are used for balance. For more of a challenge, you can slide your foot a little higher, flat against the left side of your right shin, toes pointed down. Do not place your foot against or above the knee, but just below. Hold for a few breaths. Then exhale, and return

your foot to the floor. Repeat on the other side. If seated, sit with your back straight and gently lift one foot at a time.

3   Cow: Start on your hands and knees in a table-top position, your back parallel to the floor. Keep knees directly below hips and align wrists, elbows, and shoulders perpendicular with the floor. Look towards the floor in a neutral position. Inhale and lift your chest and buttocks towards the ceiling so that your stomach moves towards the floor. Lift your head to look straight ahead. On an exhale, return to table position. To do this pose seated, inhale and bring your hands behind your back and intertwine your fingers, palms together. Exhale. Inhale again, and lift your arms gently, pulling the shoulder blades towards the spine. Gently tilt the head back and raise your gaze as you open the chest. Exhale, and release hands to neutral.

4   Cat: From cow pose or table position, exhale and tilt the pelvis back as you round the spine and drop your head. You can move between cat and cow pose, inhaling into cow, and exhaling into cat. For a seated variation, inhale and intertwine your fingers in front of you, palms together. On the exhale, rotate the wrists and push palms outward, rounding the spine and tucking the chin towards the chest.

5   Head-to-Knee: Start in a sitting position on the floor with your legs extended straight out in front. Bend your right knee, sliding your right foot into your pelvis area. Your shin stays horizontal with the floor, and your knee will move to the side. Inhale, lengthen the spine upward. Imagine there is a string attached to the top of your head pulling you up Exhale, bend your torso towards your extended left leg, reaching your arms out to your left foot. Only stretch as far as is comfortable. Hold for a few breaths and complete the pose on the other side.

6   Knee-to-Chest: Lie on your back with legs extended and arms at your side. Inhale. On the exhale, bend your knees and place your hands under your knees, drawing them gently towards your chest. Inhale while re-extending arms and legs to starting position. From a sitting position, bend forward on the exhale, and wrap your arms around your knees.

7   Downward Facing Dog: From a table position, curl your toes and press down through your hands as you lift your knees and hips up. Your spine should remain neutral. Bend the knees if your spine begins to round or shoulders move over wrists. Widen the space between your hands if the neck is uncomfortable. Hold for a few breaths.

Sacral Chakra: Opening Hips and Pelvis

1   Hip Circles: In a standing upright position, bend your knees slightly and gently rotate your pelvis in a circle, starting small and then gradually working towards larger circles. This movement is similar to using a hula-hoop. Your head and shoulders should remain upright and facing forward.

2   Pelvic Rock: Lie on your back with your knees bent in front of you. Slowly rock your pelvis up and down with each inhale and exhale. After each exhale, lift your pelvis slightly off the ground, extending the arch of your back towards the floor. You can also practice tilting the pelvis from a seated position.

3   Forward Bend: Stand upright with your feet parallel and big toes touching. Exhale, and bend forward from your hips, not your waist. Extend your arms in front of you and reach for your toes. Keep knees straight but not locked. Cross your arms so that each hand is holding the opposite elbow. If you are able, you can grab your ankles or the floor. See if you can deepen the pose on each exhale. Hold for a few breaths, and then come up slowly, one vertebra at a time. From a seated position, lengthen the spine on an inhale. Exhale, and fold forward at the hips, keeping the spine long. Reach your fingers towards the floor and hold for a few breaths, then sit up slowly.

4   Half Sun Salutation: From mountain pose, sweep the arms up and over your head. Elongate the spine. Exhale and sweep the arms back down into forward bend. Inhale, and only come up half-way, keeping the back straight. If standing, the back will be parallel to the floor. You can rest your hands on your legs as you lift the chest and look forward. Exhale back down. You can do several more half-ups, or return to neutral on the next inhale.

5   Butterfly or Bound Angle: From a seated position on the floor, exhale and bring both feet into your pelvis area, pressing the bottoms of your feet together. Let your knees fall on either side. Inhale and lengthen your spine, pulling shoulder blades back. You may fold forward on an exhale, bending at the hip and keeping your spine long, or stay neutral.

6   Open Angle: Sit on the floor in an upright position with your legs extended in front of you. Gently slide your legs to either side so that they form roughly a 90-degree angle. Rotate each leg out so that your knees point up. Stretch through your heels, and walk your hands forward through the middle of your legs. Bend from your hips and reach forward, extending your stretch on each exhale. Hold for a few breaths. From a seated position, open your knees to form the 90-degree angle, and bend through the hip, bringing your torso through the knees on the exhale.

7   Goddess Pose: Stand upright with your feet a little wider than shoulder-width apart. Angle your feet outward and gently bend your knees so that they bend above but not past the ankles. On an exhale, bend into a squat position that feels comfortable. Lift and extend your arms out to form a T-shape with your torso. Then bend your elbows and raise your forearms so that your arms resemble a field-goal shape. To engage these pelvis muscles while lying down, you can lie on your back with your knees bent. Then gently allow your knees to fall to either side, stretching your inner thighs.

Solar Plexus Chakra: Core Strengthening and Stretching

1   Seated Twist: Inhale and move your right arm behind your torso, bringing your right hand either to the chair behind or your right buttock. Place your left hand on your right thigh and lengthen the spine. Exhale, and gently twist your torso to the right. Twist your lower spine first, and then through your shoulders and head. Breathe. Deepen the twist on the exhales if you feel comfortable. Your arms are just for support. Do not pull through the twist with your arms, but engage your core. Inhale and come back to neutral. Repeat on the other side. This pose can also be done on the floor.

2   Elbow-to-Knee Twist: From a seated position. Bring your palms together in front, and bend your elbows so that your forearms are parallel to the floor. Breathe. On an inhale, bring your right elbow to your left knee. Your right forearm is now perpendicular to the floor. Exhale. Inhale, and return to center. Then bring the left elbow to the right knee.

3   Seated Side Angle: Inhale and lengthen the spine and reach both arms above your head. Exhale, and bring your right hand down the floor or seat bottom next to you and enter a side bend to the right. Keep your shoulder square and spine straight. Look up to your left arm and exhale. Inhale and return to center. Take a few breaths. On another inhale, sweep arms above again and this time bring the left arm down. Lean into a left side bend, and look up to the right arm. Exhale and return to center.

4   Revolved Abdomen: Lie on your back and gently bring your knees into your chest. Extend your arms on either side to form T-shape with your torso, palms facing up. Exhale, and send your knees to the right, keeping your back flat against the floor. Stretch through your left arm and twist your torso to the left, the opposite direction as the knees. Keep the lower back stable by drawing spine inward, you can place a folded blanket there for support if needed. Hold for a few breaths and then gently come back to neutral and repeat on the other side.

5   Boat: Sit in an upright position on the floor with your knees bent in front of you and feet flat on the floor. Place your hands on the floor just behind your hips, with your fingers stretched towards your feet. For support, you can begin by holding the backs of your legs instead. Lean back slightly, but keep spine and shoulders straight and engaged. On an exhale, bend the knees and lift your feet off the floor so that your thighs are approximately 45 degrees from the floor. Shoulder blades are pulled into the spine and core is engaged. Spine remains long and neutral. Extend your legs if able, and reach your arms forward, parallel with the floor. Hold for a few breaths. You can lift one foot at a time if more support is needed, or raise just shins to be parallel with the floor. This pose can be modified for a chair exercise by lifting the legs with knees bent.

6 Bow: Lie on your stomach on the floor with your hands relaxed at your sides. Bend your knees so that your feet rise towards your buttocks. On an inhale, arch your back and lift your neck and chest slightly. Pull your shoulders back, and reach for your ankles if flexible enough. Hold for a few breaths. For a chair exercise, sit at the end of your chair, and reach your arms to grab the back of the chair near your bottom.

7 Bird Dog: Start in table position, hands and knees on the floor, with your back straight like a table and parallel to the ground. Extend your right arm forward, parallel to the floor. Exhale and extend your left leg straight back. If it feels comfortable, lift your left leg slightly up from the floor. Pelvis and back remain parallel to the floor. As you come out of this pose, first lower your foot, then bend your knee back into table position, and lastly bring your hand back to the floor. Repeat on the other side.

Heart Chakra: Chest Openers

1 Arm Movements:

   a Arm Circles: Stretch your arms out to either side so they are perpendicular with the ground. Rotate your arms in small circles, gradually increasing the size of the circles. Switch directions and repeat.

   b Vertical Arm Raises: Inhale, and raise your arms up in front of you and above your head. Exhale, and lower.

   c Horizontal Arm Raises: Extend your arms horizontally to make a T-shape with your torso. Inhale, and bend the elbows to bring your fingertips together in front of your chest. Exhale, and extend back to T-shape.

   d Serving Arms: Hold your arms out in front of you, extended, and with palms up. Exhale, and send your arms to either side, keeping your arms straight and parallel to the floor. Opening the chest and bringing the shoulder blades back.

2 Crossed Hug: Cross your arms in front of you so that each hand is holding the opposite elbow. Slowly move your hands up your arms towards your shoulders if you can. Squeeze your arms. Notice how it feels to hug yourself. Gently release and cross arms the opposite way.

3 Half Wheel: Stand or sit upright and place hands on your lower back. Your palms against your back, and fingertips pointed down. Gently bend backwards as much as is comfortable, and allow your neck to lift naturally, chin towards the ceiling.

4 Bridge: Lie on your back with your knees bent and arms at your sides. Slowly lift your hips off the ground, raising your chest and broadening your shoulders. Hold for a few breaths if able. You can also raise your arms up and over your head synchronized with breath.

5   Cobra: Lie with your stomach on the floor. Bring your arms under your body, palms on the floor and elbows bent so that upper arms are parallel with torso. Inhale, and gently lift your head and spine, elbows still bent. Hold for a breath and gently come back down.

6   Upward Facing Dog: Lay with your belly against the floor and palms underneath your shoulders. Tops of the feet are resting against the floor. On an inhale, lift the torso up and off the ground as you straighten your arms. On an exhale, lower back down. For a chair exercise, grip the seat of your chair on either side of your thighs and gently lean back at the hips. Do not strain your arms, but use them only for balancing support.

Throat Chakra: Neck Stretches

1   Neck Stretches: Sit or stand upright with your feet flat against the floor and your chest lifted. Coordinate movements with breath and stop where there is resistance.

    a   Drop chin to chest. Inhale, move chin toward one shoulder. Exhale, chin back to center.

    b   Chin up, parallel to the floor. Inhale and rotate to the side. Exhale, return center.

    c   Left ear to left shoulder and return center. Same on the right side.

    d   Neck rolls: lift your head up from your shoulders and slowly roll in a counterclockwise or clockwise motion. Only stretch as much as is comfortable, and then move your head in the opposite direction. If you feel tightness, stop and let it relax.

2   Chin Tucking: Start in a sitting or standing position. Notice any tension in your neck. Tuck chin down and pull head up and back, as if making a double chin. Keep your eyes looking forward. This pose counters head protruding forward and rounded shoulders, like the posture many have while working at computers (Spence, 2021).

3   Fish: Lie with your back on the floor and knees bent. Inhale, lift your pelvis slightly so you can place your hands below your buttocks. Rest your buttocks on the backs of your hands, and hold your forearms and elbows near your torso. Inhale, press your arms into the floor and bring your shoulders together to lift your torso and head off the floor. Let your head fall back to reach the floor, throat to the ceiling. Breathe.

Brow Chakra: Deep Relaxation

1   Savasana (Corpse Pose): Lie on your back on the floor, with legs down in a relaxed position. Your legs should be about shoulder-width apart, and arms at your sides with palms facing up. This pose should feel natural and comfortable. Close your eyes and practice slow, deep

breaths as you relax into the pose. This pose is traditionally used for a meditation at the end of a yoga class.

2   Easy Pose (Sitting Crossed-Legged): Cross your legs at your shins, so that each foot is underneath the opposite knee. Bring your legs in towards your body and relax your feet, with their outer side against the floor. Lay your hands palms up in your lap or palms down on your knees. Sit as long as is comfortable. If you practice this pose regularly, alternate the cross of your legs on different days.

3   Child: Start from a kneeling position, with the tops of your feet flat against the floor. Sit on your heels with your big toes touching. Stretch your knees apart to hip-width. On an exhale, bend forward so that your torso comes down between your thighs. Try to bring your chest to your knees, and rest your forehead on the ground if able. Extend your arms and hands against the floor, stretching in front of you, palms on the floor. Arms can alternatively be beside the torso with fingers pointing behind you. A block or folded blankets can be placed under the hips, and between the shins to ease tension on the knees. If uncomfortable, you can widen the knees and bring the toes together to lengthen the spine. You do not need to be sitting on your heels. Hold and rest as is comfortable. If you cannot do this version of the pose, try laying on your back and bringing your knees to your chest.

4   Pigeon: Start in a table pose. On an exhale, move the right knee forward and to the right, behind your right wrist. Angle your shin so that your right foot is in front of your left knee. Rest the right shin and foot on the mat, and extend your left leg straight back. Left knee, thigh, and shin are resting on the mat. Spine is upright and engaged, hips are square. Elongate on inhale, bend forward at the hips on an exhale. Breathe. Release pose by extending arms and placing palms against the floor. Push the torso up on an inhale and return to table position. Repeat on the other side.

Breath

The cycle of breath is primal and fundamental to all aspects of life. Breath also connects individuals with their larger ecological context through the exchange of oxygen and carbon dioxide (Rama et al., 1976). Conversely, when breath is stifled or constricted, so too is the flow of one's interaction with their environment. The breath cycle is therefore key in all meditative practices. Focusing on breath helps cleanse the mind and body, and promotes sensory control and calm concentration.

Similar to posture, one's rate and rhythm of breathing signals the state of their mental experience. Breath is not under the exclusive control of either the mind or the body, but rather, can be regulated by both autonomic and conscious control. Psychological states further modify breathing patterns, and breathing habits impact mental activity in return. Due to this relationship, breath can be used as somewhat of a "barometer for levels of stress and fatigue" (Gordon et al., 2019, p. 27). During a calm state, breathing is relaxed and steady, while various emotional states produce distinct variations. While breathing patterns vary with each individual, people generally tend to hold their breath, speak as they inhale, or hyperventilate when experiencing anxiety, while they sigh and speak at the end of the exhale with depression (Bakal, 1999). This "breath language" is akin to body language, and communicates one's experience within their environment (Rama et al., 1976). It is often difficult and unproductive to seek control over thoughts and feelings, but control of breath allows for regulation of these mental activities. From an ACT perspective, the goal of breathing techniques is to allow the breath to be fluid and flexible, rather than controlled. Rather than forcing a deeper breath, aim for an effortless breath that follows the body's natural rhythm.

Deep and slow-paced breathing helps regulate sympathetic nervous system arousal (e.g. heart rate, breathing rate, blood pressure, temperature) and modulates pain perception (Chen et al., 2017). Additionally, breathing techniques are easy to learn, require limited cognitive processing, and have essentially no risks or negative side effects.

Diaphragmatic Breathing/Complete Breath

Diaphragmatic breathing uses the contracting of the diaphragm muscle to push air downward through the body, producing a relaxing and stabilizing effect on the autonomic nervous system. During a normal breath, the chest moves up and down, while the abdomen moves out and in. These movements are controlled by diaphragm and the external intercostal (rib cage) muscles underneath the ribs. To learn whether you are a chest or belly breather, place one hand on your chest and another on your stomach. Chest breathers will notice their chest and shoulders rise when they inhale, while their stomach either does not move or goes inward. Belly breathers will alternatively notice that their chest and shoulders will hardly move on an inhale, but their stomach will extend outward, and then inward on an exhale. Chest breathing is designed to be used as a back-up for the diaphragm; a supplementary emergency mechanism that increases the amount of oxygen ingested into the body to gather additional energy for fighting off a threat. As chest breathing is meant for self-preservation or escaping danger, this form of breathing tends to elicit related emotions, such as fear or anxiety. This type of breathing actually triggers a stress alarm, while learning to initiate diaphragmatic breathing can often help restore balance and a natural rhythm (Bakal, 1999).

Natural movement of the diaphragm with breath facilitates a free and coordinated exchange of energy between the primal energy of the lower chakras and the more inspired energy of the higher chakras (Rama et al., 1976). The breath moves down into the lower belly on the inhale, and then rises through the rib cage, lungs, chest, throat, and nostrils on the exhale, engaging each of the chakras. The breath should feel relaxed and effortless. If someone has developed a habit of chest breathing, this may initially feel awkward and take practice to develop a natural rhythm.

Diaphragmatic breathing is referred to in yoga as a "complete breath", and is done through only the nostrils rather than the mouth (Ajaya, 1976). A popular variation is "square breathing," often used as a behavioral health intervention. During a "square breath", the individual inhales, holds breath, exhales, and pauses for four seconds each (Rama et al., 1976). Others inhale and exhale for four seconds each, and take only a one-second pause to hold breath and between breaths. To further promote present moment attention, practice thinking "here" on each inhale, and "now" on each exhale.

Other Breathing Techniques

In Hatha yoga, breath control (pranayama) is used to stabilize breathing and produce relaxation. Pranayamic breath control involves three key processes: 1) extending exhale (approximately twice as long as inhale) to slow down the breath; 2) breathing through the diaphragm; and 3) adding resistance to each breath, such as alternating between nostrils (Chandra, 1994). Breathing exercises may be especially useful for balancing the heart chakra, as these techniques engage the chest and respiratory system, and grounding through the root chakra. Breathing techniques that engage different parts of the body (e.g. stomach, throat, nose) facilitate healing in the associated chakras.

1   Victory or Ocean Breath: With the mouth closed, practice slow, deep breaths through the nostrils. Then play with constricting your throat so that your exhale breaths produce a slight snoring or rushing sound, like ocean waves. Breath through your diaphragm. This technique may be especially beneficial for balancing the sacral and throat chakras.

2   Bellows Breath: Take rapid, diaphragmatic, forceful breaths at a pace of about 20–30 breaths per minute, combined with contraction of stomach muscles. This is done through inhaling and exhaling rapidly through the nose, while the mouth is kept closed. Inhales and exhales are the same short length. Alternate taking a few bellows breaths with normal breathing. One variation is the Breath of Fire, which emphasizes only the exhale. With this technique, the individual uses their stomach muscles to push the air from their lungs. These techniques engage the solar plexus chakra.

3   Sighing Breath: Breathe through your diaphragm, and on the exhale make an audible sigh. You can add arm movements, up on the inhale and down on the exhale to engage more of the body and the heart chakra.

4   Lion's Breath: Hold your hands up like paws and spread your fingers wide or place hands on your thighs. As you exhale, look up and make a breathy "ha" sound while sticking your tongue out. This technique promotes throat chakra energy.

5 Bumblebee Breath: Take a slow inhale, and then on the exhale close your lips tightly and make a gentle humming noise. You can also use your index fingers to gently close your ears. You can feel the vibrations on your lips. You can experiment with different humming noises and notice what sound may be most calming or energizing for you. This breath most engages the throat or brow chakras.

6 Alternate Nostril Breathing: Place a hand in front of your face, palm facing towards you, so that your index and middle fingers are between your eyebrows. Place your ring and little finger against one nostril, and your thumb on the other. Using your fingers to close one nostril at a time, take several breaths through only one nostril. Then close that nostril, open the other one, and take several breaths through only that nostril. A variation of this technique is to breathe in through one nostril and then out for the other. For example, breathe in through the left while holding your right nostril closed. Then close the left nostril, open the right, and exhale through the right. This technique may be most helpful for balancing the brow chakra.

References

Ajaya, S. (1976). *Yoga psychology: A practical guide to mediation.* The Himalayan International Institute of Yoga Science and Philosophy of the U.S.A.

Anderzén-Carlsson, A., Lundholm, U. P., Köhn, M., & Westerdahl, E. (2014). Medical yoga: Another way of being in the world—A phenomenological study from the perspective of persons suffering from stress-related symptoms. *International Journal of Qualitative Studies on Health and Well-Being, 9,* 1–10.

Bakal, D. (1999). *Minding the body: Clinical uses of somatic awareness.* Guilford.

Büssing, A., Ostermann, T., Lüdtke, R., & Michalsen, A. (2012). Effects of yoga interventions on pain and pain-associated disability: a meta-analysis. *Journal of Pain,* 13(1), 1–9.

Chandra, F. A. (1994). Respiratory practices in yoga. In B. H. Timmons & R. Ley (Eds) *Behavioral and psychological approaches to breathing disorders* (pp. 221–232). Plenum Press.

Chang, D. G., Holt, J. A., Sklar, M., & Groessl, E. J. (2016). Yoga as a treatment for chronic low back pain: A systematic review of the literature. *Journal of Orthopedics & Rheumatology,* 3(1), 1–8.

Chen, Y., Huang, X., Chien, C., & Cheng, J. (2017). The effectiveness of diaphragmatic breathing relaxation training for reducing anxiety. *Perspectives in Psychiatric Care,* 53(4), 329–336.

Defrin, R., Riabinin, M., Feingold, Y., Schreiber, S., & Pick, C. G. (2015). Deficient pain modulatory systems in patients with mild traumatic brain and chronic post-traumatic headache: Implications for its mechanism. *Journal of Neurotrauma,* 32, 28–37.

Emerson, D., Sharma, R., Chaudhry, S., & Turner, J. (2009) Trauma-sensitive yoga: Principles, practice, and research. *International Journal of Yoga Therapy,* 19 (1), 123–128.

Field, T. (2009). Progressive muscle relaxation. In *Complementary and Alternative Therapies Research*. (pp. 97–101). American Psychological Association.

Ghoncheh, S., & Smith, J. C. (2004). Progressive muscle relaxation, yoga stretching, and abc relaxation theory. *Journal of Clinical Psychology*, 60(1), 131–136.

Ginzburg, K., Tsur, N., Karmin, C., Speizman, T., Tourgeman, R., & Defrin, R. (2015). Body awareness and pain habituation: The role of orientation towards somatic signals. *Journal of Behavioral Medicine*, 38, 876–885.

Gordon, T., Borushok, J., & Ferrell, S. (2019). *Mindful yoga-based acceptance & commitment therapy*. Context Press.

Hofmann, S. G., Sawyer, A. T., Witt, A. A., & Oh, D. (2010). The effect of mindfulness-based therapy on anxiety and depression: A meta-analytic review. *Journal of Consulting and Clinical Psychology*, 78(2), 169–183.

Kiecolt-Glaser, J. K., Christian, L., Preston, H., Houts, C. R., Malarkey, W. B., Emery, C. F., & Glaser, R. (2010). Stress, inflammation, and yoga practice. *Psychosomatic Medicine*, 72, 113–121.

McCallie, M., Bloom, C., & Hood, C. (2006). Progressive muscle relaxation. *Journal of Human Behavior in the Social Environment*, 13, 51–66.

Peper, E., & Lin, I. (2012). Increase or decrease depression: How body postures influence your energy level. *Biofeedback*, 40(3), 125–130.

Rama, S., Ballentine, R., & Ajaya, S. (1976). *Yoga and psychotherapy: The evolution of consciousness*. Himalayan Publishers.

Salmon, P., Lush, E., Jablonski, M., & Sephton, S. E. (2009). Yoga and mindfulness: Clinical aspects of an ancient mind/body practice. *Cognitive and Behavioral Practice*, 16, 59–72.

Smith, J. C., Amutio, A., Anderson., J. P., & Aria, L. A. (1996). Relaxation: Mapping an uncharted world. *Biofeedback & Self-Regulation*, 21, 63–90.

Spence, J. (2021). *Trauma-informed yoga: A toolbox for therapists*. PESI Publishing & Media.

Zeidan, F., Martucci, K. T., Kraft, R. A., Gordon, N. S., McHaffie, J. G., & Coghill, R. C. (2011). Brain mechanisms supporting the modulation of pain by mindfulness meditation. *Journal of Neuroscience*, 31, 5540–5548.

8   Self-Integration

The path to self-actualization becomes confused in the presence of an underdeveloped or disorganized sense of self. Limited self-concepts and internal inconsistencies are self-perpetuating, and instinctive attempts to reconcile discrepancies can further cause self-alienation. People may reject or alter parts of themselves or experience in order to maintain a particular self-story. In this way, the actualizing tendency can lead to actions that work against true actualization when the direction of self-development is determined by self-conceptualizations rather than the true Self. Disrupted energy in the chakra system creates incongruence that results in self-discrepancies and inflexible self-concepts, while one way that COACT aims to restore energy balance is through enhancing self-development and self-integration.

The Self and Pain

Chronic pain impacts not only how individuals interact with the world, but also how they understand their sense of self. Individuals may develop mental and behavioral habits centered around managing their pain so much that they experience their identity as connected to their pain. They devote a large amount of time and energy to pain management and these habits and pain-avoiding strategies are reinforced over time. Eventually, these habits become the individual's automatic response pattern and are interpreted as their personality. In this way, their pain experience has come to define their self-concept. Importantly, pain interference with social roles and personal identity significantly influences one's ability to cope effectively with chronic pain (Harris et al., 2003).

Three categories of self-related processes have been identified in chronic pain patients: 1) a sense of self based on self-evaluation ("evaluative"); 2) a sense of self based on attributes or self-descriptions ("descriptive"); and 3) a sense of self that is detached from either of the other two categories ("contextual"). Negative self-evaluations have been particularly linked with reduced functioning, while a contextualized or transcendent sense of self is associated with improved functioning (Yu et al., 2015).

DOI: 10.4324/9781003251293-9

Researchers have used self-discrepancy theory as a framework for understanding the mechanisms through which chronic pain contributes to a compromised sense of self (Kindermans et al., 2011). Self-discrepancies elicit negative emotional experiences and occur when an individual's current self (i.e., actual self) is perceived as different from the person they believe they should be (i.e. ought self) or the person they want to be (i.e. ideal self). Self-discrepancies in the context of chronic pain may present as conditional beliefs about the self based on the presence of pain, also termed self-pain enmeshment. For those with chronic pain, self-discrepancies are associated with poor pain adjustment and greater pain interference, emotional distress, lack of pain acceptance, and psychological inflexibility (Kwok et al., 2016). The strength of pain-related self-discrepancies may predict how much the individual accepts their pain experience and the hurting or compromised self (Kindermans et al., 2011).

The relationship between chronic pain and self-discrepancies appears to be partially mediated by psychological inflexibility and the ability to flexibly redefine one's self-concept according to changing contexts (Kwok et al., 2016). This means adaptively expanding one's sense of self to accommodate new experiences. In the context of pain or somatic symptoms, this may involve recognizing a physical limitation without fusing with it. Consider three ways an individual might respond to the observation that running exacerbates their pain. One individual might react to this limitation with anger or frustration and attempt to push through the pain and continue running. Another might give up running or physical activity altogether so as not to increase their pain. A third option might be to accept this limitation and modify one's exercise routine to try running for shorter periods of time or walking. The first two responses reflect attachment and inflexibility, while the third response is an example of accepting pain, modifying goals and expectations, and expanding the self to integrate one's present experience while also moving in a values-based direction.

Self in Pain vs. Self Experiencing Pain

In the context of somatic distress, there is a distinction between the self in pain and the self experiencing pain. The self *in* pain is an example of self-as-content, and represents self-pain enmeshment or fusion. When pain becomes one's point of reference, the individual is unable to view their pain or self objectively. Pain avoidance similarly stems from an overidentification with one's pain experience, and then rejecting this aspect of the self. With the experience of the self in pain, one's awareness is filled with pain-related sensations, thoughts, and emotions. Their experience is also consumed with control-based pain management strategies (avoidance), and a conceptualized self-concept based on pain. The individual has absorbed their pain experience into their identity, such that there is no "I" unattached to their pain. The limited self-conceptualization is also maintained by a desire to avoid emotional pain and painful self-awareness associated with a traumatic or stressful event. People sacrifice contact with the stable transcendent Self and other self-perspectives as they reject the part of the self that is hurting. Rather they cling to self-stories that perpetuate pain avoidance. Lastly, as individuals limit their actions to avoid pain and lose contact with the true Self, they also lose contact with their central values. Figure 8.1. illustrates awareness of the self in pain, and the disconnection from one's true Self and values that occurs when pain consumes and dictates one's experience.

The alternative is the self *experiencing* pain, which maintains contact with the transcendent Self. From this perspective, the self is like a container with pain inside it. There is a clear differentiation between the self and pain experience, and the place of observation is distant and detached. Figure 8.2. illustrates the expansion of the self and awareness to include all aspects of one's pain and experience in order to restore connection with the body, self, and values. Everything is within the circle of awareness, and all boundaries are open.

ACT treatments do not target increasing positive self-evaluations or resolving self-discrepancies, but rather focus on expanding one's self-awareness with compassion and detachment (acceptance and defusion). With this awareness, people release the struggle with their experience and are free to direct attention towards values-based and effective action (Yu et al, 2015).

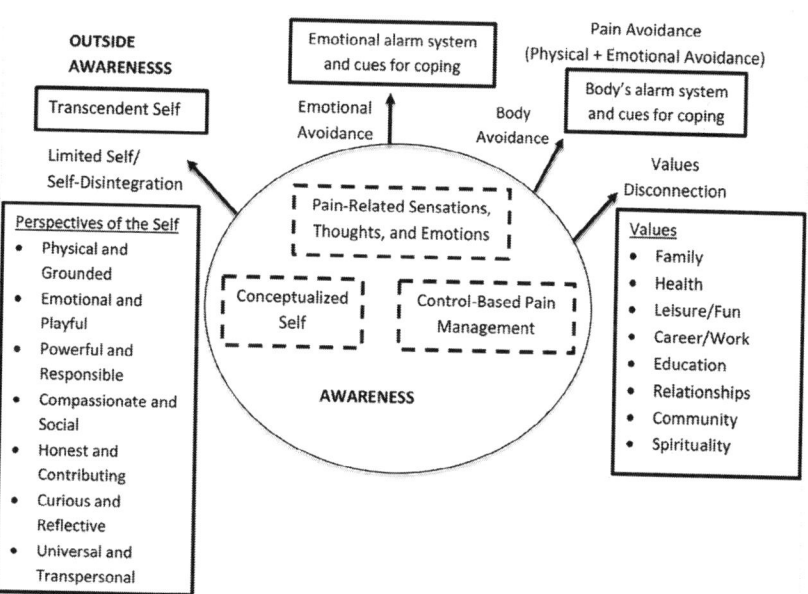

Figure 8.1. The Self in Pain

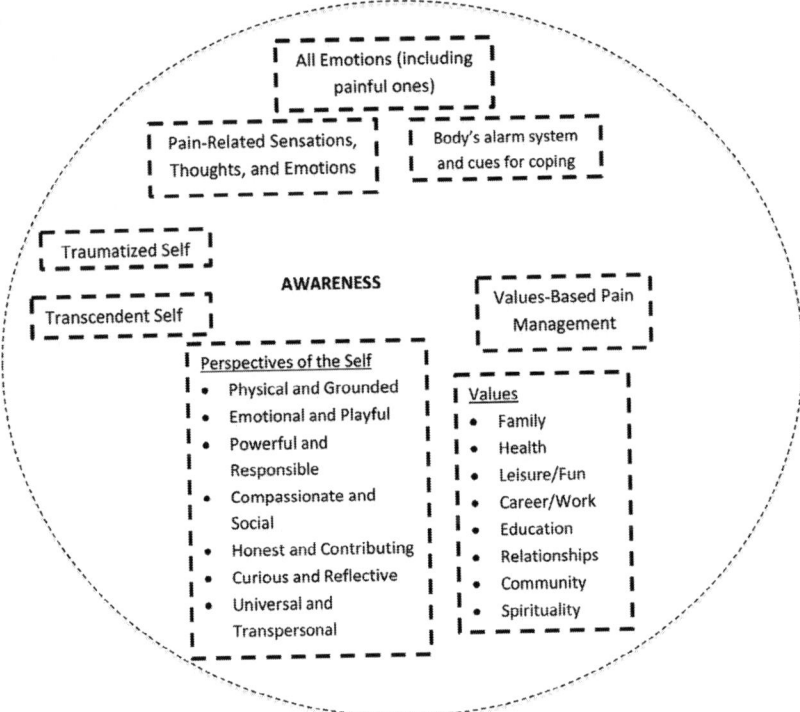

Figure 8.2. The Self Experiencing Pain

Interventions

There are numerous methods for promoting self-integration, but four key processes include releasing rigid self-stories (self-as-content), developing general perspective-taking skills, expanding the self to make room for all experiences (self-as-context), and contacting the transcendent Self. In COACT, the self-as-context exercises are further contextualized to increase flexibility of the self and self-acceptance at the level of each chakra.

Defusing from Conceptualized Selves

1   Observing Self-Stories: Bring awareness to some of your different selves. Imagine how you might describe yourself in various situational contexts (e.g., during a job interview, at a party, on a date, with your mother). Each of these selves is "true," and yet flexible and changing (the self at work, the self with family, the self with friends, the struggling self, the generous self, etc.). Practice noticing and then releasing attachments to each of these narratives. Observe how no self-story holds true in every context (Strosahl et al., 2012). To further raise awareness of the transcendent self, ask, "Who

is doing the observing?" This stable perspective is defused from the contents of experiences and able to observe self-stories without becoming entangled in them (Hayes et al., 2012).

2   Who are You?: In yoga, one develops their self-concept, or "I-ness", by repeatedly asking the simply stated but loaded question, "Who am I?" (Rama et al., 1976). This process is similar to the ACT intervention of repeatedly asking "Why?" to help patients reveal their values (Hayes et al., 2012). If one can continue to provide a justification or "reason", the core value has not been identified yet. Similarly, if the self-definition demonstrates an external attachment, such as a personality label, character trait, social role, etc., it is not reflective of one's true Self. The goal is to peel back the layers of automatic and culturally conditioned responses that often make up one's external personality in order to reveal one's true Self. The clinician can ask the patient or the patient can ask themselves, "Who are you?" Most initial responses will be a form of self-description or self-evaluation. Thank the mind for that response and ask again until one reaches, "I am me."

3   I am/I am Not: Identify two positive attributes or qualities you possess and one negative trait. For all three consider is this trait true all the time? Are there any exceptions? To foster defusion, think of specific examples in which your behavior supported each statement and when your actions contradicted each statement. Consider the functions of these self-stories, and what it would mean if they were not true. Who would you be without these stories? (Hayes, 2019).

General Perspective-Taking

Perspective-taking interventions can be any strategies that promote flexible thinking and exploring different vantage points. In general, these techniques encourage the individual to shift their perspective across persons, place, and time.

1   Words of Wisdom: Are you familiar with A Christmas Carol? You might recall that Scrooge is visited by the ghosts of Christmas past, present, and future. I want you to imagine you are similarly taken to view a version of yourself in the past. What age of yourself do you go visit? Why that one? What do you recall about being that age? What events were going on or what were you navigating at the time? What were your goals and dreams back then? What does this say about your values? Hold this image of yourself clearly in your mind. How does it feel to observe yourself at this age? Now imagine this past self could speak to you now. If they could see what your life looks like and your current actions, how would they feel? Which of your present actions would this self wish were different? Which would they be excited about? What does this say about your values?

Alternatively, imagine you are whisked away to the future. Assuming you continue on your current trajectory, what is your future self like? What are they doing? What is important to them? How do you feel about this future self? Is it who you want to be? If not, what could you do differently now to change your path? How does it feel to look at your present self from this perspective? Would your future self say there is anything for you to learn from your current situation? What guidance might they offer for your current actions? Which of your current actions would they be glad or grateful you are doing? Which actions might they suggest you change? What does this say about your values? (Hayes, 2019; Strosahl et al., 2012).

2 Adopting Another's Perspective: Experiment with trying on a different perspective by mentally placing yourself into the shoes of another person. Try to place your awareness behind the eyes of someone else and see the world as they do. It can be someone you know or someone fictional. Do you have someone in mind? Tell me about this person. Who are they? What is important to them? What are their goals? What are their challenges? What thoughts, feelings, sensations, or memories might help or hurt them in pursuing their values? How do they interact with others? How does it feel to be this person? What do you like or not like about this perspective?

3 Talking to A Friend: Imagine you are talking to a friend who is going through all the same experiences that you are right now. How would you feel as you heard about their situation? What would you want to say to them? What would you want for them? How would you feel towards them?

4 Movie/Book Metaphor: Try to picture the story of your life as either a book or a movie. What chapter or scene are we currently in? What might be the name of this chapter or scene? As the audience, how do you feel about your character at this point? What would you hope the character does next? What do you want the character to learn from this part of the story? Remember that your life is more than just this chapter. Recall some previous chapters, and reflect on how the story has evolved or changed (*Rewriting Your Story*, Hayes, 2019).

5 Changing the Genre: What type of book/movie is this story? How would you categorize the genre? How could you tell this story from the perspective of a different genre?

6 Chapters of Life: Imagine the chapters of your life story are categorized by theme. Some chapters might be, "Favorite Days," "Goals and Dreams," "Hurts and Heartbreaks," or "Growing Pains." You might not read through the book in a sequential order, but flip back-and-forth between chapters. When an event occurs, think about which chapter this experience might go in your book. The hope is to honor all chapters and make room for each and every experience.

7 What Could This Be?: This exercise helps reduce functional fixedness by increasing thought flexibility (Hayes, 2019). Start by picking any

object in the room. Now think about all the different ways you can imagine using that object. Allow your mind to come up with silly, obscure, or even bizarre possibilities. Anything goes. You can make a list or you can just say them as they come to you. Try not to hold back. See if you can think of at least ten different ideas.

This exercise can be applied to somatic symptoms. As an example, suppose a patient presents with a dull pain in their lower abdomen and some mild nausea that comes and goes. Ask the patient, "What could this be?" Perhaps the patient ate too much or something their body is having difficulty digesting. One's mind might even think of more serious medical conditions like appendicitis or diverticulitis, but what else could it be? Maybe the patient is anxious about an upcoming presentation at work, stressed about planning their child's birthday party, or remembering their favorite aunt that passed away. Could it also be that their stomach is actually a small ocean, and the waves are causing discomfort? Maybe somehow their abdomen got filled with Silly Putty? Try to think of the most absurd explanation you can imagine. Again, the goal is to increase flexibility and practice expanding perspectives. Some patients may provide ideas that increase anxiety, such as serious medical conditions. The goal of this exercise is simply to generate as many possibilities as they can. Allow the patient to offer these ideas, and then also help them come up with additional silly responses or opposite extremes.

8   Chessboard Metaphor: Imagine yourself standing on a huge chess board. Think of it as stadium-sized, with giant towering pieces. If you are familiar with the Harry Potter movies, think of the chess scene in the Sorcerer's Stone where the characters can ride the large chess pieces. The pieces on the board represent your thoughts, feelings, and sensations. You might label the pieces on one side of the board the "good" ones and the other side the "bad" ones, and assume that one side is going to win as the game is played. You select a "good" game piece, climb aboard, and brace yourself for battle. From this perspective, the contents of your mind seem much larger than you and you are fighting against parts of yourself. Each side then takes turns making a move. However, the more you fight and play the game, the harder the game becomes. Suddenly you realize there are an infinite number of pieces, so even if you manage to remove a few "bad" pieces from the game, new ones only take their place. From this perspective, you feel helpless, exhausted, and certain of eventual defeat. What if you were not on the chessboard with the piece? Is there another perspective? Some patients may have the idea that they are one of the players, but the player still maintains an investment in the outcome of the game. The board, however, is not attached to who wins or loses, it simply holds the space. The same metaphor can be applied to various sports where the patient is encouraged to take the perspective of the field/court rather than the ball or players (Hayes et al., 2012).

Contextualizing/Expanding the Self

Energy disruption within each chakra contributes to lost contact with certain perspectives of the self. To integrate or re-integrate these selves, individuals can experiment with consciously adopting these self-perspectives. The process is similar to imagining the perspective of another in order to build empathy and compassion. However, instead of placing one's awareness behind the eyes of another person, they place awareness within part of the self that has been lost, rejected, or underdeveloped. Each chakra also governs a particular emotional experience that must also be accepted and integrated into the self. See Table 8.1 for a summary of the self-perspectives and emotional experiences associated with each chakra. The Self-Integration Outline (Appendix I) can help patients clarify aspects of their self-story they want to let go, parts of the self they want to contact and bring into awareness, and specific actions they will take to build connection with the desired self-perspective.

Root (Physical & Grounded Self): Engaging the self in the root chakra involves connecting with the body and movement; as well as grounding awareness in the here and now to build a sense of stability and make room for fear.

1   Strong Body: Bring your awareness to your current physical sensations. You may use somatic awareness techniques (mindfulness, yoga, muscle relaxation, deep breathing) to facilitate communication with the physical self. As you observe your body's sensations, what thoughts or feelings show up in the mind? How does your mind view the body? Is the mind critical of the body for having pain? Does the mind get frustrated or upset with the body for these sensations? Does the mind view the body as causing problems? Now shift your awareness actually into your body, rather than observing your body from the mind's perspective. You might imagine your body is personified, now a separate entity with thoughts and feelings. How might the body respond to the criticisms of the mind and being treated like the "bad guy"? How does it feel to be thought of as weak and problematic? What does the body want the mind to know? Listen with compassion to the body's expression. How much is it hurting? What does it need?

Table 8.1 Chakras and Self-Perspectives

	Root	Sacral	Solar Plexus	Heart	Throat	Brow
Self-Perspective	Physical & Grounded	Emotional & Playful	Powerful & Responsible	Compassionate & Social	Honest & Contributing	Curious & Reflective
Emotional Experience	Fear	Guilt/ Blame	Shame/ Anger	Jealousy/Resentment & Grief	Doubt/ Judgment	Depression/ Despair

What is the body trying to communicate? Imagine the body could speak to the mind. It might say something like, "I know you are hurting. I am hurting too" or "I am carrying a lot right now, and need your help." Listen to the body's struggle and needs. Rather than viewing the body as the enemy or part of the problem, try to see the body as a member of your team. Hear the body's strength in asking for help.

2   Thank the Body: Take a moment to express gratitude for all the things your body does for you. It might not feel like your body is on your side right now, but take a moment to reflect on that. What are some of the actions your body performs that you are thankful for? What is going right? What is your body doing for you at this moment? Thank your body for each breath you take. Bring your awareness to each of your senses, and thank the body for that experience. Imagine going through your day and thank the body for each action it allows you to perform. Hold gratitude and appreciation for all the organs, muscles, and systems in the body that give life and allow you to move through the world.

3   Facing Your Fear: Recall a time in which you felt really afraid or scared. This could be a recent event or experience from your past. How did that fear feel? Describe what was happening in your body and mind. Can you picture yourself in that moment? Now see if you can take the perspective of this fear. What was your fear trying to do? (e.g., protect you). What does this say about your values? As you bring your awareness into the self experiencing fear, ask, "What does this self need?" Fear stems from feeling a lack of safety or security. What does the self experiencing fear need to feel safe or secure? Acknowledge the need and the hurt associated with this unmet need.

4   Inner Safe Space: Recall a time in which you felt safe. Where were you? Who were you with? What were the circumstances? If no memory comes to mind, think of a favorite place in a movie or book, or even a place of your own imagination. Think of a place where you would feel free to be yourself, where you would feel safe to explore, and where you would feel relaxed enough to rest. What might this place look like? How does it make you feel? Pull up that feeling of safety and notice where you feel it in your body. Do you notice any warmth or relaxation? Make this memory more vivid by adding detail. Fully immerse yourself in this place of safety and groundedness.

5   You Belong Here: Call up a feeling of fear. Allow your experience of fear to enter your awareness. Notice where you feel that fear in your body. Notice any muscle tension or changes in your breath or heart rate. Take a few breaths and continue to hold this feeling. How does it feel to invite fear into your awareness? As you notice any tension or

anxiety show up, observe and welcome these sensations. Greet any anxious thoughts with kindness. To each thought, feeling, memory, and sensation, experiment with saying, "you can be here." How does this feel? If this is comfortable, you can experiment with saying "you are welcome here" to each anxious thought or sensation. Even further, try saying "you belong here." Notice how each step feels as you shift from tolerating your fear, to accepting and even embracing it. Notice what happens to your fear as you try these different experiments.

Sacral (Emotional & Playful): Connecting with the self in the sacral chakra involves giving up the search for control and exploring the world with playful excitement. This aspect of the self also needs emotional acceptance, and for feelings of guilt and blame to be integrated.

1   Laugh at Yourself: Being silly and laughing helps to build flexibility and defuse from rigid self-stories. Think of some of your favorite comedy movies. You can probably recall several comedies in which the humor stems from a series of disasters and plans not coming together. As an audience, we laugh as we watch the characters struggle in these ridiculous situations (e.g., *Meet the Parents, Bridesmaids, The Hangover)*. Now think of a time in your own life that felt chaotic and stressful. When it felt like one event after another seemed to not go as planned or did not meet your expectations. Did you try to gain back control only to find that the harder you tried, the more mess was created? Imagine you are watching these events play out like a movie. Take a moment to observe your own actions and find the humor. Laugh at your attempts to control the uncontrollable, and the strange ironies and coincidences that make life so unpredictable.

2   Let's Play: During times of stress, people often become hyper-focused on trying to control and manage the problem. Opportunities for fun and play are often given up to focus on the problem. Imagine yourself as a child or think of a child you know, and notice how this child plays. What does that look like? How does a child experience the world? See through their eyes and feel that sense of adventure and excitement. Can you recall a time in which something ordinary was turned into a game? Perhaps you used boxes to build a fort or made your chores into a race. How did it feel to immerse yourself in the game? Now imagine this child approaches you and asks, "Will you play with me?" How does that feel? What do you want to say? Do you tell the child you are too busy or have more important things to do? How would that make the child feel? What would it feel like to say yes?

3   Embracing Emotions: Picture yourself as a knight, sworn to protect the kingdom. Right now your emotions feel like monstrous creatures trying to invade, and you must fight. One at a time you strike them down or manage to tie them up, but then another comes from a new direction.

Allow yourself to sit with this feeling of mental and physical exhaustion. You are fighting and fighting, but another monster can always be seen headed right towards you. Now imagine these "monsters" are actually trying to help you. They are messengers from throughout the kingdom and trying to provide you with important information. How does this realization make you feel? How might you want to approach these creatures differently? How might you try to communicate with them?

4   Room for Regret: Nobody acts in accordance with their values all the time. Think about some of the choices or experiences you feel guilty about. As you do this, make room for your guilt, regret, hurt, and any other associated emotions. See if you can hold these painful emotions with acceptance, recognizing that it is okay to have these feelings. Now reflect on what your feelings of guilt say about your values? What is it that you care about that has caused you to feel this pain? What can you learn about what is important to you? Now see if you can remember the person you were back then. Place your awareness behind the eyes of the you that made those choices or lived through those experiences. What thoughts or feelings were in your mind at the time? What was the context of these experiences? Imagine you are looking at the self who made the choices you regret. Is this person hurt, sick, tired, or otherwise struggling to care for themselves? Do their choices maybe "make sense" given this context? Is it possible that your past self did the best they could with the resources and information they had at the time? You might tell yourself something like, "I wish that had not happened, and it's okay that it did" or "I would have wanted to make a different choice, and I did the best I could." You can hold your guilt with acceptance or you can release your guilt.

5   Alignments: Can you think of someone or a character that shows great discipline and has difficulty letting loose? (e.g., Captain America, Superman, Spock). What do you think it's like to experience the world in this way? What are the benefits and challenges? Now think of a character that is care-free, pleasure-seeking, and/or tends to rebel against others' rules (e.g., James Kirk, Iron Man, Indiana Jones). What is this experience like? What are the benefits and challenges? Which do you see yourself more as? Which would you like to be more? Why?

Solar Plexus (Powerful & Responsible): The solar plexus self holds one's strength of will and personal power. Connecting with this self involves honoring one's autonomy while defusing from unhelpful thoughts to make room for feelings of shame and anger.

1   Captain Response-Able: Experiences of stress and pain can leave individuals feeling powerless over circumstances outside their control. Imagine yourself as a superhero. What qualities do you have? How does this feel? What do you do when faced with a challenge? Do you take action? What might happen if you hesitated or did nothing?

Even when the situation is dire and the clock is ticking, a superhero always seems to find a way to respond. The outcome is not always ideal. Buildings may be destroyed, and lives may even be lost. But the point is that they always *do* something. They try their best to make a positive impact even in desperate situations. You have this same ability. No matter the context, there is always something you can do. You might come up with a mental image or physical pose that reminds you of this superpower. For example, you might stand tall with your hands on your hips in a Superman pose to facilitate bringing awareness to this self-perspective. You might also imagine putting on your superhero cape or mask. In moments where you start to feel powerless, imagine becoming this superhero self and getting ready for action.

2   Just Trying to Help: The mind is a natural and expert problem-solver, but this can sometimes backfire. The mind will engage in problem-solving strategies even when no problem is present. The mind will look for problems just so it can solve them! The mind might even start to think that the Self is a problem that must be "solved." This is not helpful at all, but the mind is doing its job. Have you ever tried to help someone that did not need or want any help? Perhaps you offered a suggestion only to be shut down, told to go away, or even aggressively snapped at. How did that feel? You were just trying to help, right? Alternatively, have you ever received terrible advice from someone who meant well? Has anyone offered to help you when you knew that person would only make the task more difficult? How did you respond? When the mind offers unhelpful thoughts, perspective-taking skills can help us remember the mind is just doing its job. Thank that mind for trying to be helpful, and let that thought go. We can appreciate the mind's sincere attempts to help, and also not accept its advice.

3   Choose Your Character: Imagine you could create your own character for life like in a video game. What qualities would you want them to possess? How would you want them to interact with others? What would drive them? What goals would they pursue? Now imagine how it would feel to really take on this persona, to walk through life as this character. You can! Just like in a video game, you cannot always choose the context or situations you encounter, but you can always choose how you respond.

4   Facing the Bully: How might you feel about someone who is being bullied? Sometimes our mind is like a bully. It gives us self-critical thoughts that make us feel bad or ashamed. Imagine you are a bystander who witnesses the mind being a bully. You could argue with the bullying thoughts, but they would only argue back and get louder. Defusion helps to dismiss the bullying mind's comments as meaningless. You take power back from the bully by not buying into the bully's words (Strosahl et al., 2012). Now how do you feel about the person being bullied? How might you offer support or comfort to the self that has been bullied by the mind?

5   Anger Shield: Anger is a secondary emotion triggered by a desire to feel powerful or cover up more vulnerable feelings, such as sadness or hurt. When situations make us feel small or threatened, anger helps us feel strong and capable. Recall a time in which you felt angry. Was your anger trying to protect you or someone you love? Was your anger protecting your rights or something else you care about? What does your anger say about your values? Think of a time in which you were angry, and allow that experience to fill your body and awareness. Where do you feel that anger? As you notice these sensations in your body, imagine the feeling of anger building a shield around you. As a shield, your anger is meant for defensive actions, not offensive. Notice what this shield is protecting you from. Express gratitude for this protection. Then notice if this shield disconnects you from anything. Does this shield also keep something positive from being near you? How would you know when to put down this shield?

Heart (Compassionate & Social): Integrating the self in the heart chakra encourages compassion and empathy for oneself and others, was well as accepting feelings of jealousy, resentment, and grief.

1   Heart-to-Heart: Experiences of trauma and stress can cause emotional pain that close off the heart for self-protection. Being emotionally cut-off from others leads to internal conflict regarding a longing for connection and beliefs that one is better off on their own. Closing off relationships also means the individual does not have the opportunity for corrective experiences to learn how to build and maintain healthy relationships and positive connections. Take a few moments to bring awareness to your heart. Notice the rhythm of your heart and pace of your breath. On each exhale, imagine your heart expanding slightly (like the Grinch from Dr. Seuss's *How the Grinch Stole Christmas*). Feel the energy in your heart soften and relax. Gently invite your heart to a conversation. Imagine your heart is an old friend you have not spoken with in some time. A lot has happened in their life since you last connected. Witness the hurt the heart has endured and offer validation. You might say something like, "I see all that you have been through" or "I understand why you don't let people get too close." Invite the heart to share what it feels. Listen with compassion.

2   Puppy Love: How does a dog love? Does their love have to be earned? Are there rules for their love? Does their love come and go? How does it feel to be loved by a dog? A dog is a great example of unconditional love and being fully present in the moment. See if you can take this perspective of a dog. Look at yourself through a dog's eyes. Try to experience that delight and enthusiasm for you just being you. How do you think you could hold this love for yourself? How can you show yourself this kind of love?

3   Bigger or Bitter? Feelings of resentment are like poison to the heart, and jealousy has often been termed the "green-eyed monster" for how it can consume an individual. Can you remember a time you felt jealous? Why were you jealous? Was there something you wanted or needed? Was it something someone else had? When these feelings show up, first observe and acknowledge them. Notice how this feeling shows up in your body, and what need is lacking. Are you upset because you are missing something you need, or upset because someone has something you do not think they deserve? Take a moment to notice how this jealousy has affected you. How does it feel in your body? How has it affected your relationships? How does it consume your experience? How would it feel to release this feeling? Then ask yourself, "Do I want to be bigger or bitter?" You have the choice to carry your resentment or to expand the Self and make room for this experience with greater compassion.

4   Enough for Everyone: Oftentimes we experience jealousy and resentment out of a false sense of scarcity. From a limited perspective, we believe that someone else's gain is our loss. To expand your awareness, imagine you are sitting at a table and someone brings you a plate of food. You are very hungry but there is only a little bit of food on your plate. You start to eat slowly, hoping to make it last as long as you can. Then someone comes over with their own plate of food and sits down next to you. You immediately notice there is more food on their plate than yours. You are annoyed, but try to let it go. Then someone else comes over and sits on your other side. Their plate is heaping full. You feel cheated. They try to make friendly conversation with you, but you are too distracted by your hunger and frustration. How come they got more? Staring at your plate only increases your resentment. After seeing a few more people sit down with plates full you decide you have had enough. You eat what is left on your plate and get up to leave without saying a word to anyone. On your way out the door you pass a table full of food. You realize there is a buffet, and everyone is helping themselves. You were so worried about what you were given and what everyone else had, that you never even looked around the room! There is enough for everyone.

5   Love & Loss: The pain of grief can sometimes be so intense and overwhelming that we feel our heart simply cannot take it. It is common for people to try to push these feelings outside of awareness and criticize themselves when these feelings show up. Remember, we hurt where we care, and the more we care, the more we hurt. One way to make room for this pain is to acknowledge this expression of love. Some individuals have the thought, "It happened so long ago, I should be over it by now!". I often ask my patients, "Have you stopped loving the person that has passed?", which often prompts a confused glance. "Of course not!" is usually the response. The source of distress is not the grief itself, but the fight to suppress or get rid

of one's grief. Hold your feeling of grief for a moment. Remember the person or object you have lost. Feel the love you have for them. You might feel some sadness or pain as well, and this feeling is an indication of how much you care about the person you have lost. Hold that feeling of love. Would you be willing to stop caring about this person if it meant you would not feel grief?

Throat (Honest & Contributing): Connecting with the self of the throat chakra involves authentic self-expression, and making room for emotions that interfere with meaningful action (doubt, judgment).

1   Court Stenographer: Imagine you were tasked with making an objective record of your mental activity. This means noting your thoughts, feelings, memories, etc., exactly as they are. Like a court stenographer, your job is to record these experiences without judgment or evaluation. You can practice by actually writing down notes or taking mental notes. Remember, your job is to keep an unbiased and complete record. This includes honestly recording even unwanted thoughts and feelings. Defusion strategies can also be used to remember thoughts are just thoughts, and feelings just feelings.

2   The Overheard Conversation: Imagine you overheard someone speaking to another person exactly the way your mind speaks to you. How do you feel about the language this person uses? What kind of energy are they putting out? How do you feel about the person speaking? How do you feel about the person they are talking to? Our words are a reflection of the energy we give out. What kind of energy do your words communicate or inspire?

3   Vocal Warm-Ups/Vocal Awareness: Listen carefully to the sound of your own voice. Notice the tone, rhythm, volume, and pitch. How does your voice change as you move through a sentence? Experiment with altering different aspects of your voice. Make your voice breathier, muffled, nasally, raspy/hoarse, harsh, resonant, sing-songy, strained, twangy, whispered, wobbly, yawny, etc. Notice how you feel when using each style. Do some make you feel stronger and bolder? Do others make you feel more shy or insecure? How does your usual speaking voice make you feel?

4   Where Do You Give?: Imagine you have $86,400 to donate or give every day. You cannot hold on to it, and it must be spent. Who do you choose to give this money to? Does it go to family or friends? Do you give some money to charities or other organizations? What do these groups do that you find meaningful? What do your choices say about your values? Each day you wake up with 86,400 seconds to use. How do you want to use this time?

5   80th Birthday: Imagine it is your 80th birthday and you are surrounded by all your family and friends. One by one, people begin to stand and

speak about your accomplishments, the impact you have had on their life and the larger community, and how you lived your life. What do you hope people will say? (Hayes et al., 2012).

Brow (Curious & Reflective): Self-integration within the brow chakra requires an openness to one's inner wisdom and bringing awareness to emotions that limit perspective and perceived freedom (depression, despair).

1   Sitting with Sadness: If your depression was something you could see in front of you, how would it appear? What colors, shapes, textures, or other qualities would it possess? Would your depression have the form of a person, an animal, or something else? You may choose to draw it. After you have generated an image of your depression, imagine sitting down right beside it. Maybe you even place your arm around it, and you just sit together.

2   Different Glasses: Have you ever tried on a pair of tinted sunglasses? You may have noticed the world can look quite different depending on the lens we are using. Imagine there is a rainbow set of glasses. Each pair is a different color and creates a different way of perceiving the world. What do you imagine the red pair does? How does the world look while wearing this pair? The orange? Yellow? Green? Blue? Purple? What pair do you usually wear? Which would you like to wear?

3   The You Behind it All: Imagine how you would describe yourself to a new acquaintance that you would like to befriend. You might start with "I am…" What if you wanted to develop a romantic relationship with this person? Now describe yourself as you would in a job interview. Next if you were picked up by the police and falsely accused of a crime. What aspects of your self-description change? What aspects stay the same?

4   General Perspective-Taking (releasing illusions/fixations, seeing from a wider angle)

  a   Words of Wisdom
  b   Movie/Book Metaphor
  c   What Could This Be?
  d   Who Are You?

5   Connecting with the Transcendent Self

Contacting the Transcendent Self

Steven Hayes (2019) offers a four-step process for connecting with the transcendent Self. First, defusion strategies are used to let go of the conceptualized self, or attachments to self-stories. Second, the individual notices the observing self (self-as-process), the self who is always present and serves as the container for our mental contents. Sometimes clinicians ask patients, "Who is doing the noticing?" to help them identify this sense of self, and may encourage them to make statements like, "I am not my thoughts or feelings. I hold my thoughts and feelings within my awareness." Third, individuals develop perspective-taking skills and seek to make these a habit. They practice shifting their perspective across dimensions of person (I/You), place (Here/There), and time (Now/Then) ("perspective-taking relations"). Lastly, they extend these perspective-taking skills to move the transcendent sense of self towards greater connection and consciousness with others. Self-stories and conceptualized selves create rigid boundaries between "I" and "not I", while perspective-taking and higher levels of consciousness expand the self and redraw these boundaries in order to reduce this separation. Self-as-context has typically been conceptualized as transcendent perspective-taking, but is now understood to also include empathy, compassion, and self-compassion (Hayes et al., 2012)

References

Bakal, D. (1999). *Minding the body: Clinical uses of somatic awareness*. Guilford.

Harris, S., Morley, S., & Barton, S. B. (2003). Role loss and emotional adjustment in chronic pain. *Pain*, 105, 363–370.

Hayes, S. C. (2019). *A liberated mind: How to pivot toward what matters*. Avery.

Hayes, S. C., Strosahl, K. D. & Wilson, K. G. (2012). *Acceptance and commitment therapy: The process and practice of mindful change* (2nd ed.). Guilford.

Kindermans, H. P., Huijnen, I. P., Goossens, M. E., Roelofs, J., Verbunt, J. A., & Vlaeyen, J. W. (2011). "Being" in pain: The role of self-discrepancies in the emotional experience and activity patterns of patients with chronic low back pain. *Pain*, 152, 403–409.

Kwok, S. S. W., Chan, E. C. C., Chen, P. P., & Lo, B. C. Y. (2016). The "self" in pain: The role of psychological inflexibility in chronic pain adjustment. *Journal of Behavioral Medicine*, 39, 908–915.

Rama, S., Ballentine, R., & Ajaya, S. (1976). *Yoga and psychotherapy: The evolution of consciousness*. Himalayan Publishers.

Strosahl, K., Robinson, P., & Gustavsson, T. (2012). *Brief interventions for radical change: Principles & practice of focused acceptance & commitment therapy*. New Harbinger.

Yu, L., Norton, S., Harrison, A., & McCracken, L. M. (2015). In search of the person in pain: A systematic review of conceptualization, assessment methods, and evidence for self identity in chronic pain. *Journal of Contextual Behavioral Science*, 4(4), 246–262.

9   Values-Based Action

Values are deeply personal and vary between individuals. One's values infuse life with meaning, fulfillment, and purpose; contributing to life satisfaction. Life satisfaction additionally enhances one's ability to cope with chronic pain (Dezutter et al., 2017) and stress (Park, 2010). Pain highlights where values have been placed. People hurt where they care, and at the center of all pain is a value, something that is loved or cared about.

Acceptance and Commitment Therapy (ACT) is the most prominent values-based treatment approach and emphasizes not only what someone does, but *how* they do it in order to establish a continuous values-driven direction. Values are not goals, objects, or desired outcomes that can be achieved or completed, but freely chosen qualities of action (Hayes, 2019). Values supply the *why* which helps determine the *what* (i.e. specific behaviors) and *how* to generate meaningful and purposeful action. For example, my desire to write this book is not a value, as this is a definable goal that I hope to complete. However, some of my values related to writing this book are holistic and compassionate healthcare, challenging myself, and contributing to the field of mind-body medicine. There are many specific actions I can perform to pursue these values, and there will always be more ways I can move in these directions.

Behavioral Experiments

Every COACT visit should conclude with the patient agreeing to try something different, a behavioral experiment. Any variation of one's usual habits is significant in terms of increasing psychological flexibility and behavioral variability. Even a minor shift reduces the inflexibility of the patient's current attachments. The behavioral experiment can be a new or varied behavior that the patient plans to practice on their own or with others, at home or in the community, or in any other context. The new behavior may be an observable action or a different way of relating to their internal events (e.g. practicing a defusion or acceptance technique). A good experimental plan is one that the patient possesses the skills, resources, and motivation to execute (Robinson, 2020). After each

DOI: 10.4324/9781003251293-10

behavioral experiment, whether the patient actually performed the behavior or not, the patient is encouraged to reflect on the experience. The hope is that each experiment allows the patient to learn something new. Did they perform the intended behavior? If so, what was that like and how did it impact the problem? If not, what were some of the barriers that made this behavior change unrealistic? The clinician must be aware of three factors in order to facilitate greater behavioral variability in their patient: 1) ensure the patient understands the intention and goals of the experiment; 2) ensure the patient feels confident in the experiment plan when they leave the visit; 3) establish a values context for the experiment such that the patient understand how the experiment connects back to their values and presenting problem (Robinson, 2020).

Behavioral experiments are a form of behavioral activation, but done in the service of values. Individuals are motivated to do more of the activities they care about and replace habits that do not help them engage with what is most important to them. Further, these variations can be specifically planned to increase behavioral responses congruent with the values of a particular chakra. A common framework for setting behavioral plans is using SMART goals (Specific, Measurable, Attainable, Relevant, Time-Oriented). This means establishing a behavioral experiment that is a specific and well-defined behavior, measurable in some way, achievable, relevant to the patient's values, and time-oriented. The Committed Action Plan (Appendix J) can be used to help patients identify specific ways they can move in the direction of their values rather than pain control.

Values-based action, or "committed action," means the pursuit of one's values, knowing that missteps will occur. After a lapse it may be helpful to ask yourself, "Did any of my values change?" If not, then recommit to your values and resume the direction of desired change (Hayes, 2019). The other psychological flexibility skills can be engaged to support values-based action. Defusion encourages distance from culturally sanctioned values and judgments about values, such as feeling the need to justify or rationalize one's values. Values are meaningful to someone simply because they choose for them to be, there are no right or wrong values. Acceptance helps individuals listen to their pain and recognize their values in their pain. Pain shines a light on what one most cares about. Presence allows individuals to stay in the moment of moving towards their values; as opposed to planning action for the future or worrying about action done in the past. Each moment is an opportunity to be aware of one's values and take another step in their direction (Hayes, 2019). This chapter will provide practical tools for generally increasing values-driven actions, as well as how to contextualize values-based action for working with each chakra. Table 9.1 summarizes a few values associated with the chakras.

Table 9.1 Chakras and Values

Root	Sacral	Solar Plexus	Heart	Throat	Brow
Family, Group Belonging, Health, Nature, Physical Activity, Order, Safety, Stability Trust, Self-Care	Adventure, Beauty, Control, Excitement/ Fun, Humor, Pleasure, Romance, Sensuality, Sexuality, Self-Gratification	Assertiveness, Challenge, Courage, Independence, Persistence, Power, Responsibility, Self-Esteem, Skillfulness, Self-Development	Compassion, Empathy, Equality, Forgiveness, Generosity, Intimacy, Kindness, Love, Relationships, Self-Acceptance	Authenticity, Community Service, Contribution, Creativity, Honesty, Humility, Industry, Integrity, Justice, Self-Expression	Clarity, Curiosity, Gratitude, Imagination, Knowledge, Mindfulness, Open-Mindedness, Wisdom, Spirituality, Self-Awareness

Conscious Action

To develop values-based habits, individuals aim to practice conscious intentionality in each action. Self-study allows individuals to observe which experiences contribute to discontent and internal imbalance, and this observation creates opportunities for learning how to restore equilibrium and maintain stability (Ajaya, 1976). It is far easier to hold a stance of nonattachment and remain focused on one's values during stressful times if one has been practicing these skills routinely. When experiencing stress, people tend to fall back on behavioral patterns that are well-rehearsed. Practicing valued actions with everyday tasks helps these habits become more automatic and accessible in any context.

Bringing awareness and intentionality into every action further helps improve efficiency. When people hurry or complete tasks while distracted, they often make mistakes that actually increase their workload. Conscious action is a "process of bringing mindfulness, greater sensitivity, awareness, and gentleness, to each and every experience" (Ajaya, 1976, p. 104). Slowing down and allowing the mind to concentrate on one action at a time enables individuals to bring themselves fully into the moment and focus all resources on the task at hand. During early adoption of this practice, people may find that when they give up their regular multitasking habits, there are simply not enough hours in the day to do everything they have been trying to do. This is another opportunity to revisit one's values, and the function and purpose behind each task. Are some of these tasks related to wants rather than needs? Are they pursuing attachments or guided by the true Self? Do these actions lead to lasting contentment or fleeting gratification? Liberating oneself from some of these "to-do" items may actually afford more time and energy to use on what really matters most.

Habit Replacement

COACT targets building habits that are aligned with the individual's authentic Self and values, while disengaging from behaviors that conflict with these values. Building values-based habits that are sustainable and self-rewarding increases the likelihood they will be continued. Small adjustments can lead to large changes over time, so it is usually best to start with a simple alteration or deviation from usual routine. This should also be something that can be immediately acted upon. One trick to building new habits is to pair desired behaviors with actions already routinely performed. This allows the established behaviors to serve as a cue for the new behavior. Another technique is habit reversal, which involves engaging in new behaviors that are incompatible with an undesired behavior (e.g. an avoidant-based strategy). The effects of habit reversal are enhanced when combined with psychological flexibility skills (Woods & Twohig, 2008).

Mantra Affirmations

In traditional yoga, a unique and personalized mantra is given to a student by their master, similar to a spiritual prescription (Ajaya, 1976). Mantras are sometimes called prayers, and serve as a focus point for meditation. They are also used to hold conscious intention around one's actions and experience. Establishing such an intention instills purpose and direction for the day, and also encourages one to reflect on how their actions align or do not align with their expressed values. This prompts re-evaluating or changing one's actions to be more consistent with their stated commitment or desire (Ajaya, 1976). For example, someone may start their day with the prayer, "Let my interactions today communicate honesty and respect towards others." They then might catch themselves later telling a white lie or making an insensitive joke to a friend. Recalling their morning prayer may encourage them to reflect on these actions and change how they speak to others later in the day. Using the same prayer daily for at least a few weeks also helps build the habit of being guided by this prayer. Often the goal is to develop values-based traits and patterns of behavior that eventually become mostly automatic. It is recommended that individuals create or choose a mantra that is contextualized to the type of connection and values-based direction they are seeking. Some examples for mantras associated with each chakra are listed here:

Root: I trust myself. I am caring for my body.
Sacral: I seek fun and enjoyment in my day. I am willing to experience all my emotions.
Solar Plexus: I choose my responses. I can handle the challenges of today.
Heart: I accept myself as I am. I will treat others with kindness and compassion.

Throat: I speak the truth. I will listen with integrity.
Brow: I am open to new ideas and perspectives. I am grateful.

General Valued-Action Interventions

1   Pain Exposure: Exposures are common behavioral interventions, used by both ACT and traditional Cognitive Behavioral Therapy (CBT). These two treatment models, however, approach exposure interventions differently. In ACT, exposures are used to help an individual alter their relationship with the object or experience causing distress and generate alternative ways of responding. The goal is not to reduce anxiety or change the experience (as in CBT), but rather learn to observe, describe, and then accept the emotion or sensation as it is (Hayes, 2019). While the exposure exercise can be limited to a particular time, situation, or emotion, the level of acceptance is all-or-none. A jump is a jump. If needed, one can start with an exposure to an emotion or sensation that is less distressing, but acceptance is "all in" (Hayes, 2019). Exposures can be done to physical and/or emotional pain, and should be done in pursuit of a valued action (Hayes, 2019). A clinician might ask the patient, "What are you willing to make room for in order to engage in activities that are important to you?" Additionally, patients can generate a list of activities or situations they avoid due to their pain, and then set behavioral experiments to intentionally engage in these activities.

2   Secret Mission: Values-based actions are inherently meaningful through their association with what matters most to an individual. When an action is performed in pursuit of one's values, the individual is not seeking any form of social approval or recognition. However, some values-based actions are likely to be admired or appreciated by others (e.g. an act of kindness or generosity, a professional accomplishment). To strengthen awareness of how fulfilling values-based behavior is for its own sake, experiment with performing a values-based action in secret (Hayes, 2019). Notice how it feels to engage in this behavior simply because you want to, and without any social reinforcement or praise. If you experience a desire to tell others about this behavior, notice this pull and reflect on what you may be needing. Experiment with smaller actions if the desire to share with others is too great, and identify actions that can be comfortably performed in secret.

3   Reducing Self-Discrepancies: Engaging in actions that are aligned with one's central values helps foster self-integration and reduce self-discrepancies. The experience of living with chronic pain can increase awareness of unsuccessful goal attainment or goal conflict due to pain (Kwok et al., 2016). Chronic pain may produce self-discrepancies through the perception of failing to meet one's hopes (actual-ideal discrepancy) or responsibilities (actual-ought discrepancy). In response

to pain, individuals may need to redefine their goals and expectations, let go of unreachable goals, and select more realistic ones (Wrosch et al., 2013). The pursuit of unattainable goals and pain avoidance are both inflexible coping styles that interfere with one's ability to effectively adapt to pain. Flexible goal adjustment can instead protect against the development of self-discrepancies and associated distress (Dezutter et al., 2015; Schmitz et al., 1996). To establish realistic and meaningful goals, the individual must be in contact with their values, which serve as a directional guide for action and increased functioning. It has further been proposed that cognitive restructuring may be the most effective strategy in matching one's actual-self to their ought-self guide, while behavioral strategies are most useful for matching one's actual self to their ideal self-guide (Boldero & Francis, 2000).

a   Setting Realistic Goals: Individuals may need to recognize and accept certain limitations due to their pain experience, and identify creative alternative means for engaging their values.
b   Cognitive Restructuring: Challenging beliefs about what the patient "should" or "ought" to be able to do helps defuse from rigid self-stories and reduce actual-ought self-discrepancies. These mental rules can be observed and released as the patient develops flexibility of thought and self-concept.
c   Behavioral Activation: Building behavioral repertoires of values-based action reduces discrepancies between the actual and ideal self.

Chakra-Based Values Interventions

Root Chakra

Values-driven actions of the root chakra engage physical activity, group bonding, and grounding.

1   Physical Exercise: Collaboratively set SMART (specific, measurable, achievable, relevant, time-oriented) goals for exercise. The key is to create exercise goals that fit the context of the patient's life. This includes their symptom presentation or pain, as well as work schedule, parenting demands, energy level, motivation, etc. It is better to set smaller goals that are more realistic and help the patient build confidence than to set larger, less achievable goals. Clinicians can help the patient identify forms of exercise they enjoy or experiment with new styles of exercise.
2   Activity Pacing: This intervention is often used in the treatment of chronic pain to disrupt the pattern of over- and underactivity. It is common for individuals to limit their activity while experiencing pain, which contributes to lost strength or endurance. Many then overcompensate by doing too much when their pain is less severe,

which can exacerbate pain levels afterwards. While stuck in this cycle, one's activity level is always determined by their pain. Pacing allows the individual to set realistic activity goals followed by rest. This rhythm is unique to each individual, and requires some experimentation to find the pace that works best for them. One can start by rating their daily pain on a 10-point scale (1 = no pain; 10 = worst pain imaginable). If their pain increases by 2 points with activity, they rest until the pain is back to the starting level. The goal is that their pain is no worse at the end of the day, even though they engaged in some activity. Encourage the patient to keep track of the time (how many minutes) they can perform an activity before their pain level rises, and how long they need to rest before their pain returns to its starting point. Once this is known, the patient can set activity goals that are time-based rather than pain-based. Patients may benefit from working on just portions of their daily routine at first, instead of trying to complete an entire task at once. For example, rather than trying to complete all the steps in cleaning a load of laundry, maybe the patient starts with just trying to gather all the dirty laundry in a basket. Within ACT, activity pacing is done in the services of values and to enhance functioning. The goal is for individuals to resume as much of their normal activity as possible. They may not perform desired actions at the same speed or efficiency as they once did, but continuously pursue a values-based direction.

3   Enjoy the Outdoors: Spending time outside and connecting with the natural world helps with grounding. Patients may go for a mindful nature walk/hike or simply sit outside and bring their awareness to the support of the chair and earth beneath them.

4   Self-Care: The needs of the root chakra are basic physical and safety needs. This includes food, water, sleep, and shelter; as well as routine self-hygiene, exercise, and rest/relaxation. Many people find it difficult to prioritize self-care and meeting these needs, especially in contexts of stress, trauma, and pain. To build self-care habits, experiment with small and simple actions at a time.

5   Family/Cultural Engagement: The root chakra is associated with one's "roots"- their familial and cultural backgrounds. Spending time with family (including one's chosen family), practicing cultural traditions, and learning more about one's ancestry are all ways to increase a sense of grounding and belonging.

6   Build Your Safe Space: One's environment has a huge impact on their sense of safety and stability. The internal environment (i.e. the mind) may adopt aspects of the external environment, such that people feel more anxious and mentally disorganized when their external environment is chaotic, messy, or dangerous. Creating a physical safe space in one's home (or elsewhere, if the home is not a realistic option) can help restore or enhance a sense of stability and

security. This space can be a small corner, a room, or the entire home. Decorate or bring in objects that make you feel safe and comfortable. Everything in the space should promote a sense of relaxation and peace. This is *your* space. For individuals with trauma, reclaiming ownership of their environment can be especially empowering.

Sacral Chakra

Values-driven actions of the sacral chakra involve emotional flexibility and exploring fun and pleasurable activities.

1   Play!: During times of stress, people often let go of fun activities. However, a life without fun or play is essentially a recipe for emotional distress. Think of activities you either previously enjoyed but have stopped doing or activities you have often thought about trying but never got around to it. If nothing comes to mind, find a list of ideas online and try a few. The Centre for Clinical Interventions in Australia offers a Fun Activities Catalog with 365 items on their website (Center for Clinical Intervention, 2019). These activities can be as simple as drawing or playing with your pets. What is important is setting time aside to do something that is purely for your own enjoyment. This may be a skill that requires practice, and that is okay! Start with smaller goals to build the habit.

2   Healthy Pleasure: Pleasure is an important part of life, but moderation is key. Both over- and underindulgence can produce negative consequences for one's health and happiness. As taste is the sensory experience of the sacral chakra, you may experiment with indulging in some of your favorite foods. Allow yourself to be completely present with the experience and the sensation on your taste buds. There is no need to consume a large quantity, but take your time and savor each bite. One could also engage the pleasure of the sacral chakra through sexual activity. What really enhances the energy of the sacral chakra is releasing any efforts to control the experience. Partnered or solo, the experience should not be forced or effortful, and there is no required outcome. Be in the moment and observe the sensations, thoughts, and feelings of the experience.

3   Choose Your Adventure: Whatever adventure means to you, plan an activity that engages your sense of excitement and exploration. Maybe you are a natural thrill-seeker, or maybe you get anxious looking out a second-story window. Perhaps just altering your usual routine in some small way (e.g. sleeping on the other side of the bed, brushing your top teeth before your bottom teeth) feels adventurous. Great, try that! Perhaps you want to skydive. That is great too! Choose how you want to experiment with adventure.

4   Silliness is the Spice of Life: The sacral chakra energy reminds people to give up control and be flexible. Experimenting with actions that make you feel silly helps breakthrough existing limitations. People feel silly when they do something outside of their usual repertoire, perhaps something they believe is ridiculous. This form of play pushes people to drop the usual rules of "serious" behavior, and actually aim for the absurd. In doing so, they may gain a new perspective on the silliness of their prior limitations. It has also often been said that "laughter is the best medicine." Empirical evidence backs this up, as laughter is associated with improved coping with pain (Dunbar et al., 2012).

5   Make Time for Romance: Making time for romance is another way to engage the sacral chakra. Romance is not synonymous with intimacy or sexual activity. Instead, romance refers to the experience of mystery and excitement in one's relationships, including their relationship with life. Romantic acts could be planning a special date night with a partner, learning about a different aspect of your partner, or making an effort to show your love and appreciation in some way. Romance further does not have to be partnered. It may be romantic for an individual to take a trip by themselves, explore a new area, or start a new passion project.

6   Treat Yourself: Moderation is key in many aspects of the sacral chakra; however, it can be nice to splurge now and again. This could be as simple as buying yourself a small coffee while you are out getting groceries. What makes this act beneficial is not how much you do or how much money you spend, but the intention you set by taking a moment to treat yourself. As you do something for yourself, pause and acknowledge this celebration of life.

Solar Plexus Chakra

Values-driven actions of the solar plexus chakra target personal responsibility and achievement, including building strengths and skills.

1   Responsible Action: Many behaviors are automatic habits that have developed unconsciously. Some are useful (e.g., brushing your teeth every night) and others are less so (e.g. having a beer every night). Becoming responsible (or response-able) involves consciously examining these habits, releasing those that do not serve one's values, and intentionally building habits that are values congruent. Track a few of your daily actions, and observe if there are some you would like to stop, increase, or keep as they are.

2   Strength Building: Personal power is a reflection of one's self-concept and self-esteem. When people recognize their own strengths and areas for growth with compassion and acceptance, they are able to demonstrate their power in a way that reflects their values and communicates

compassion and respect for others. When people feel weak or inadequate, they do not recognize the power they possess and therefore may intentionally or unintentionally misuse this power. This can lead to manipulative or aggressive behavior, or allowing oneself to be bullied and mistreated. Engaging in acts that help individuals recognize their strengths and build healthy self-esteem is therefore important for solar plexus chakra. This could be making a list of one's positive traits, engaging in activities that make them feel capable and strong, or increasing positive self-talk to remind oneself of their best qualities.

3   Go Your Own Way: Experiment with acts of independence by doing something on your own that you might normally ask someone to do with you. Maybe you go to lunch or go shopping by yourself. For some this could mean learning to drive or even moving into your own place.

4   Master It: The solar plexus is connected to experiences of ambition and achievement. Ongoing learning and skill-development builds mastery and a sense of accomplishment. Individuals can experiment with learning something new, or further their knowledge of something they already enjoy.

5   "Just Because I Choose To" (Hayes, 2019): Personal power is recognized as individuals learn they can make commitments and stick to them purely because they choose to. ACT co-creator Steven Hayes recommends experimenting with unimportant changes to highlight that people do not need a *reason* to build new habits. Individuals are often motivated by compliance, guilt, shame, fears of rejection, longing for acceptance, emotional avoidance, and other "reasons" that undermine the experience of free choice (Hayes, 2019). These experiments are not permanent changes, but may be conducted over a week or a month to demonstrate how one can build a habit for no important reason. Examples might be wearing a different color of socks, waking up a bit earlier each day, or eliminating a type of food from your diet.

6   Building Assertiveness: Assertiveness is a way of clearly and directly communicating one's thoughts, emotions, and needs, while also holding compassion and respect for others. It is the balance between aggressive and passive. Assertive communication is honest, appropriate, respectful, and direct (H.A.R.D). Learning to be assertive is not about being assertive in every interaction, but learning to practice discernment based on the situational context. Individuals can experiment with assertive action by communicating in "I statements" (e.g. "I feel…when…"), setting and holding appropriate boundaries (e.g. practice saying "no"), and explaining their feelings and choices without providing "reasons."

Heart Chakra

Values-driven actions of the heart chakra emphasize social relationships, compassion, and nurturance.

1   Social Engagement: Actions that build relationships and social engagement help heal the heart chakra. Individuals can spend an afternoon with a friend, participate in a social group, or attend an enjoyable activity where they can meet and interact with people who share their interests.

2   Acts of Kindness: Acts of kindness build a sense of connection with others and communicate care and compassion. Experiment with doing something nice for someone else. This can be a small gesture for a stranger or planning a surprise for a loved one. The size of the action is not important. The purpose is setting the intention to increase kindness in the world. For many, it is easier to share love and kindness towards others than themselves. Acts of self-compassion and kindness towards oneself also promote self-acceptance and positive energy in the heart chakra.

3   Forgiveness: Practicing forgiveness can open aspects of the heart that were closed-off. Forgiveness expands the heart to make room for one's hurt, while also choosing to move forward with values-based actions.

4   Intimacy: Open the heart by building stronger connections with others. Acts of nurturance, caregiving, and empathy all help build intimacy and a deeper knowing of someone else. This type of intimacy is not sexual or romantic (as with the sacral chakra), but aims to truly see and accept someone else exactly as they are.

5   Grieving with Love: The depth of one's grief is a mirror for the depth of their love. When grief shows up, engage in an act that communicates this love. What can you do to show love for the person that has been lost? How can you carry this memory in a loving way?

6   No One is An Island (Hayes, 2019): Individuals are more likely to keep commitments that are shared or made public. People are further impacted by the behavior of those around them, such that a behavior change made by one person becomes more likely to occur in others within their social circle. Decide on a values-based change or action you would like to perform, and include members of your social support team.

Throat Chakra

Values-driven actions of the throat chakra focus on conscious communication and integrity.

1   Sound of Silence: Much of talking is actually about the past, plans for the future, or imagined/conceptualized possibilities; all of which pull attention away from the moment. While language affords humans with a means for social communication, it also inherently creates barriers. People often over-rely on the use of words to express and connect, at times losing the richness of communicating with

nonverbals, such as facial expressions, eye-contact, and body language. Words are also used to critique, evaluate, and judge; as well as to discharge frustrations or worries, and to provide comfort (Ajaya, 1976). This is not inherently problematic, of course, but can be done in the service of avoidance rather than expression. Silence removes the distraction and defense of talking, and helps to remove the trivial aspects of communication in order to promote more authentic expression. Practicing silence helps to develop enhanced awareness and receptivity to the expression of others, allowing one to listen and receive rather than fill the space with their own personal expression. Yoga psychologist Allan Ajaya (1976) recommends experimenting with a day of silence, but you may also try shorter experiments. Choose a time where you do not have to work, but will be running errands and spending time with friends and/or family. Let these people know in advance that you are experimenting with silence, and have a brief written note ready to share with anyone else you might encounter. At the end of the experiment, reflect on your experience. What did you observe?

2   Learn to Listen: Listening with integrity is just as important as speaking honestly. Practice listening intentionally to your friends, family, and loved ones. Hear their words and the meaning they are trying to convey. Do not interrupt or be too eager to offer your own ideas. Wait until they have finished speaking. Then, thank them with sincere appreciation for sharing with you. Reflect your understanding of what they shared and ask them to confirm your interpretation.

3   Where Did You Hear That?: Where and how an individual receives information significantly impacts the content and quality of the information they receive. As this material gets absorbed, it enters the mind and sometimes even the self. The information consumed has the power to alter thoughts, feelings, and behaviors, thereby influencing one's health and wellness. Consider how you get information. Are these reliable sources? Could these sources have other motives for spreading particular information? Do you engage in gossip or speculation about topics you are not knowledgeable about? Think of the impact of this communication. How might you seek truthful and reliable sources of information? What do you want to do when you encounter someone sharing false information? What kind of information do you want to communicate and spread into your communities?

4   Make Your Mark: The throat chakra energy orients individuals towards contribution and generativity. People want to do something that will have a lasting impact or help their communities flourish. Reflect on your values and think of some way you could make a difference for something you care about.

5   Creative Expression: All forms of art and creative expression enhance the energy of the throat chakra. Perhaps you have previously enjoyed

a particular creative form that you could get back into. Maybe you want to try something completely new. Experiment with any style of creative expression. Practice defusion from any self-critical thoughts, and acceptance of feelings of doubt or uncertainty. You will never know what you could produce if you do not take that first step.

6   Conscious Intentions: Prayers or mantras can be used to state an intention or make a commitment to pursuing a particular value. Today, vision boards are popularly used for the same purpose of manifesting a desired life direction. Using mantras to set conscious intentions helps promote authentic action. Experiment with setting a conscious intention for the day in the morning, and then reflect on this experience at the end of the day. How were your daily actions guided by this intention? Were there moments where you forgot or lost sight of this intention? Were you able to refocus? How did it feel to bring this purpose into your routine activities?

Brow Chakra

Values-driven actions of the brow chakra concentrate on spiritual development and exploring new possibilities and perspectives.

1   Open Mind: The brow chakra energy is enhanced when individuals are open and curious to learn something new. As opposed to learning through skill-building, which engages the solar plexus chakra, learning at the brow chakra level is about seeking knowledge and wisdom. You could take a class or do some reading to explore new ideas and learn a different perspective. You might also have a conversation with someone with different beliefs, and be open to learning something you did not know or think about before.

2   Meditation/Mindfulness: Practicing mindfulness or meditation develops the brow chakra. Consider creating a routine and consistent practice for at least a few weeks to enhance self-awareness and observation skills.

3   Journaling: Journaling is a popular practice for coping and self-reflection. What you journal about is of less importance than taking the time for self-reflection. You may reflect on the day you have had, the day ahead, something that happened long ago, your hopes for the future, your feelings about something, etc. Experiment with setting a schedule for journaling to help build the habit. This could be dedicating a few minutes at the beginning and/or end of each day, or anywhere else you tend to have some free time.

4   Spiritual Practice: All practices of spirituality, faith, or religion engage the brow chakra. Whatever faith or philosophy you subscribe to, reflect on the ways you practice your spirituality or how you could include aspects of your spirituality into your daily life.

5   Gratitude: Gratitude can be practiced in a multitude of ways. You could make a gratitude list or simply take a few moments to reflect on all that you are grateful for. See if you can even practice gratitude for some of your pain. Are there lessons in your pain that you are grateful for?

6   Perspective-Taking: Building habits of perspective-taking and self-as-context skills particularly engage values associated with the brow chakra (e.g., curiosity, open-mindedness, imagination, wisdom). Develop behavioral patterns that reflect flexible perspective-taking and practice self-as-context exercises, such as those described in chapter eight.

References

Ajaya, S. (1976). *Yoga psychology: A practical guide to mediation.* The Himalayan International Institute of Yoga Science and Philosophy of the U.S.A.

Boldero, J., & Francis, J. (2000). The relation between self-discrepancies and emotion: The moderating roles of self-guide importance, location relevance, and social self-domain centrality. *Journal of Personality and Social Psychology*, 78(1), 38–52.

Centre for Clinical Intervention (2019, May 11). Information sheets – depression. https://cci.health.wa.gov.au/Resources/For-Clinicians/Depression.

Dezutter, J., Luyckx, K., & Wachholtz, A. (2015). Meaning in life in chronic pain patients over time: Associations with pain experience and psychological well-being. *Journal of Behavioral Medicine*, 38, 384–396.

Dezutter, J., Dewitte, L., Thauvoye, E., & Vanhooren, S. (2017). Meaningful coping with chronic pain: Exploring the interplay between goal violation, meaningful coping strategies and life satisfaction in chronic pain patients. *Scandinavian Journal of Psychology*, 58, 29–35.

Dunbar, R. I. M., Baron, R., Frangou, A., Pearce, E., van Leeuwen, E. J. C., Stow, J., Partridge, G., MacDonald, I., Barra, V., & van Vugt, M. (2012). Social laughter is correlated with an elevated pain threshold. *Proceedings of the Royal Society B: Biological Sciences*, 279(1731), 1161–1167.

Hayes, S. C. (2019). *A liberated mind: How to pivot toward what matters.* Avery.

Kwok, S. S. W., Chan, E. C. C., Chen, P. P., & Lo, B. C. Y. (2016). The "self" in pain: The role of psychological inflexibility in chronic pain adjustment. *Journal of Behavioral Medicine*, 39, 908–915.

Park, C. L. (2010). Making sense of the meaning literature: An integrative review of meaning making and its effects on adjustment to stressful life events. *Psychological Bulletin*, 136, 257–301.

Robinson, P. J., (2020). *Basics of behavior change in primary care.* Springer.

Schmitz, U., Saile, H., & Nilges, P. (1996). Coping with chronic pain: Flexible goal adjustment as an interactive buffer against pain-related distress. *Pain*, 67, 41–51.

Woods, D., & Twohig, M. P. (2008). *Trichotillomania: An ACT-enhancement behavior therapy approach workbook.* Oxford University Press.

Wrosch, C., Scheier, M. F., & Miller, G. E. (2013). Goal adjustment capacities, subjective well-being, and physical health. *Social and Personality Psychology Compass*, 7, 847–860.

10 Case Examples

Three fictional case examples are presented to demonstrate the evaluation and intervention strategies presented in this text. Each case example illustrates a unique presenting symptom, different method for assessing the patient's chakras, and contextualized intervention ideas for targeting somatic awareness, self-integration, and values-based actions.

Case #1: Courtney

Courtney is a 26-year-old black female. She has a diagnosis of fibromyalgia, and her symptoms include fatigue, back pain, tingling in her hands and feet, headaches, poor concentration, and difficulty falling asleep. She also reports a depressed and anxious mood, and she worries about her physical health.

Evaluation

Contextual Interview: Courtney lives with a close friend. She has a distant relationship with her parents, who live a few hours away. Courtney always felt her mother was overly critical of her, and her father was not home much due to working multiple jobs. The family struggled financially when Courtney was growing up, and Courtney can remember sometimes going to school without breakfast or lunch. Her 21-year-old brother lives with their parents, and they have a good relationship. Courtney moved to a large Northeastern city to attend college, and stayed after graduating with a bachelor's degree in English. She identifies as bisexual, and recently went on a third date with a woman she is excited to get to know better. Besides her roommate, Courtney has a small group of close friends she sees at least weekly. Courtney works as a waitress and enjoys her job, but it is physically demanding and can be stressful. She enjoys reading, listening to music, and watching baking shows. She shares that she would like to learn how to bake and cook someday. She drinks alcohol three nights a week (two to four drinks per occasion), and smokes marijuana with friends about once a month. She does not smoke cigarettes or use any nicotine products.

DOI: 10.4324/9781003251293-11

It sometimes takes her a few hours to fall asleep. She worries at night, and sometimes her back pain makes it difficult for her to get comfortable. She eats at work during most of her shifts, which involves mostly fried and high carbohydrate foods. Her primary care provider has encouraged her to lose weight. She is on her feet at work, but otherwise has no regular exercise.

Problem Context: Courtney's symptoms started around age 20. She was in college and working two jobs when she started having frequent headaches and muscle aches. These progressively worsened and she was diagnosed with fibromyalgia at age 22. She reports that her symptoms tend to be worse when she is stressed, when her sleep is particularly poor, and when visiting her parents.

Stress Evaluation: Courtney rates her current stress as a six out of ten. She would like to pursue a career that involves writing, but is not sure where to start. She worries about paying her bills and always feels like she is trying to "catch up." Her parents do not know she is bisexual, and Courtney worries how they would react to this. Last week a customer at work directed a racist comment towards her, and she is still angry thinking about it. She rated her childhood stress as a seven, largely due to financial strain and poor relationships with her parents. She shared that the family always had financial stress, but especially after Courtney's grandmother died when she was nine. They had a close relationship, and Courtney's grandmother often provided childcare and financial support for the family.

Workability: Courtney reported she spends a lot of time watching television or reading in bed when not working. On her days off, she usually feels too tired to do much. Her friends often invite her out, but she declines. She has noticed that they seem to be inviting her less often now. Courtney notes that despite resting in bed, she does not feel better the next day. She has been gaining weight within the past year, and is worried about her health. She would like to have more energy to spend time with her friends and maybe attend a yoga or exercise class.

Chakra Assessment: The clinician decides to use the Circle of Pain Assessment to organize information about Courtney's pain and pain management strategies, as well as self-perspectives and values that she is disconnected from. See Figure 10.1 for Courtney's Circle of Pain Assessment.

Clinician: "To help us better understand the bigger picture of your symptoms, I would like to try an exercise together. The circle in the middle represents what you currently allow in your awareness. It is natural to try and push experiences of pain outside of awareness, but sometimes we also end up pushing out parts of ourselves and activities that are important to us. We may find we threw out some 'good' with the 'bad.' This map will help us visualize what else has maybe been pushed away as you have tried to manage your symptoms."

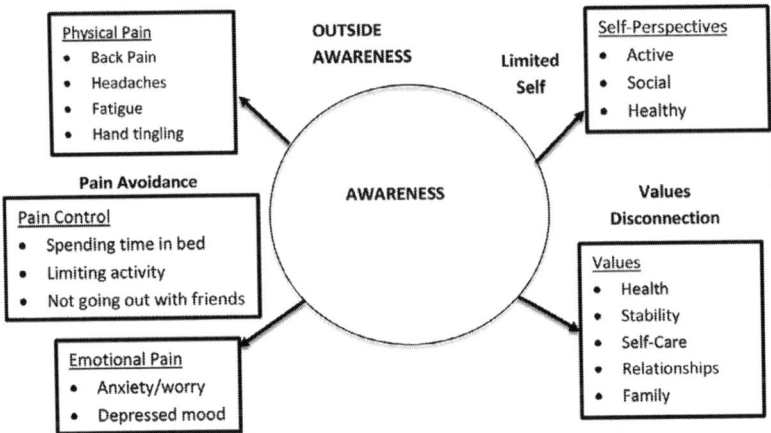

Figure 10.1 Courtney's Circle of Pain Assessment

Problem Reframe

Clinician: "It sounds like your pain and fatigue make it difficult for you to live the life you desire. To manage these symptoms, you have tried resting at home when you are not working. However this comes at the cost of not spending time with your friends and being more active. You are worried about your physical health, and would like to find ways to care for yourself. Am I understanding that right?"

Courtney: "Yeah, that pretty much sums it up. I definitely think my biggest problem right now is my health. I feel really out of tune with my body, and I want to lose weight. I just do not know where to start."

Treatment

Looking at Courtney's Circle of Pain Assessment, issues of the root chakra are most apparent (e.g., back and hand pain; anxiety; lost contact with from healthy and active self-perspectives; disconnection from values of health, stability, self-care, and family). Some concerns related to the heart chakra (e.g. social perspective and value of relationships) and brow chakra (e.g. headaches, depressed mood) are also present. Given that Courtney expresses feeling particularly disconnected from her body, somatic awareness exercises that engage the root chakra may be a helpful starting intervention. The second intervention example is creating a behavioral plan to increase physical activity, aligned with Courtney's values of physical health and self-care. This could be done during the same visit as the somatic exercise or a following visit.

Tree Pose

Clinician: "It sounds like tuning into your body may help us learn more about what your body needs and what its limits are. We call this developing somatic awareness. Just like any other new skill, the more we practice somatic awareness, the easier and more natural it will feel. There are several ways we can bring our attention to the body. Some of the methods I use most are muscle relaxation, breathing techniques, and yoga postures. Does one sound more interesting to you?"

Courtney: "I have been wanting to try more yoga, so maybe that one."

Clinician: "Okay, great. Would you feel more comfortable trying this exercise seated or standing?"

Courtney: "I guess I can try standing."

Clinician: "Okay, we will stand together. If you change your mind and prefer to sit, let me know. To start, I invite you to stand with your back straight and feet parallel. We will take a few breaths together. (Practice one to three slow diaphragmatic breaths). We are going to try something called Tree Pose. After your next breath, lift your right heel, coming onto our right toes. Rest your right heel against your left ankle. Find a fixed point on the wall to focus your attention to help with balance. If you feel comfortable, you can also try lifting your foot further so that your foot is flat against your shin. Let's breathe here. (Practice one to three slow diaphragmatic breaths). Now we will do the same on the other side. Gently place your right foot back to the floor, and we will lift the left heel. Rest it against your right ankle. (Practice one to three slow diaphragmatic breaths). Now we return to a neutral standing position. What do you think of that exercise? What did you notice in your body?"

Courtney: "I notice that I feel more relaxed and my feet feel stronger. It was hard to keep my balance at first, but then it got easier. I also kind of wanted to close my eyes."

Clinician: "You can absolutely close your eyes if you prefer, and I am glad you noticed that it got easier as you did the exercise. The goal is not necessarily to feel any particular way during or afterwards, but to practice bringing your attention into your body and observing whatever sensations are there. Do you think you might be able to practice at home?"

Courtney: "Sure, I think it might be nice to practice before bed, maybe even when I wake up."

Mindful Physical Activity

Clinician: "You have mentioned that getting more exercise and improving your physical health is important to you. I wonder if it would be helpful for us to talk about setting some realistic goals to move in the direction of this value."

Courtney: "Yeah, I think that would be helpful. I get so overwhelmed whenever I try to exercise, and then just give up."

Clinician: "It can be really hard to build new habits and make changes. Sometimes our mind gets excited and wants to do too much at once. Let's focus on setting goals that are realistic and achievable for you right now."

Courtney: "Okay, that sounds good."

Clinician: "Alright, so do you have any ideas for what kind of physical activity you most enjoy or would like to try?"

Courtney: "I guess I like going for walks. Does that count?"

Clinician: "Absolutely! Walking is a great way to get the body moving, and enjoy the outdoors. How often do you think you could realistically go for a walk?"

Courtney: "Hmm...maybe twice each week. I would like to say more, but I am not sure I would do it."

Clinician: "I think that sounds like good self-awareness. My hope is to set you up for success, so I want these goals to feel manageable. We are also building these self-care habits, so we can start small and then increase the goal later if you feel ready. How long do you think each walk could be?"

Courtney: "I think at least 30 minutes."

Clinician: "That sounds like a good start. Are there days of the week or times of day where you think going for a walk fits your schedule best?"

Courtney: "Yeah, I think before work on Tuesdays and Thursdays would work."

The clinician helped Courtney create a specific plan to engage in a values-based action. To further engage the root chakra with somatic awareness, the clinician could provide education on mindful walking and encourage Courtney to observe her body's sensations as she walks.

Case #2: Mateo

Mateo is a 43-year-old Hispanic male. He presents with recurring stomach pain, nausea, and acid reflux. He has also been diagnosed with irritable bowel syndrome.

Assessment

Contextual Interview: Mateo lives with his wife of 15 years and their three children (ages 14, 11, and 6). His relationship with his wife has been recently strained due to stress. Their 14-year-old son has struggled with the transition to high school, and is failing several classes. Their 6-year-old was also recently diagnosed with ADHD. Mateo has held the same factory job for 12 years. He used to enjoy it, but now has a co-worker that belittles Mateo in front of the other staff and uses a racist Hispanic accent when speaking to Mateo. Mateo's parents immigrated to the United States from Chile before Mateo was born. His mother lives ten minutes away and he sees her often. His father passed away four years ago. Mateo had a distant relationship with his father due to his father's heavy alcohol use.

When Mateo was a child, his father would often be angry and belligerent while drinking. Mateo recalls one time that his father shoved him to the ground for being in his way, and another time that his father threw a bottle at the door. His father would be verbally abusive while intoxicated, calling Mateo "stupid" and "useless." Mateo enjoys spending time with his children, but does not have any specific hobbies. Mateo generally sleeps well, but sometimes wakes up in the night and has difficulty falling back asleep. He reports eating a fairly healthy diet, but has been eating less due to his stomach discomfort. He used to enjoy working out, but has not felt well enough to exercise for several months. He smokes a half-pack of cigarettes each day and drinks about 36 ounces of coffee in the mornings. Mateo typically drinks two to three times in a month, but in the past six months he has been increasing his alcohol use. He is now drinking at least four days each week, and consumes three to five beers on each occasion. He denies any other substance use.

Problem Context: Mateo's stomach pain started about two years ago. The pain is present most days, and every day that he works. The pain sometimes improves when he gets home, but is worse if he and his wife argue. He recalls having stomach aches often as a child, and that he thought he "grew out of it." He recognizes the pattern between his symptoms and stress, but also worries he might have a serious medical condition. Medical testing has not identified any other diagnosis.

Stress Evaluation: Mateo rates his current stress as a seven out of ten, and his childhood stress as a five. He is worried he might lose job due to taking many sick days. Mateo also shares that his relationships with his wife and children have been stained lately, which has exacerbated his stress.

Workability: Mateo is currently managing his symptoms with increased alcohol use and reduced food intake. His medical provider has told him that alcohol is likely worsening his symptoms, but Mateo says it is the only thing that helps him relax. He feels ashamed of his alcohol use, particularly because of how alcoholism impacted his father. He and his wife have also been arguing about his alcohol use. Mateo is spending less time with his family due to stomach distress, and is worried about getting fired due to missing so much work.

Chakra Assessment: Mateo's prominent somatic symptom is stomach pain, suggesting dysfunction in the solar plexus chakra. He also shares feeling dissatisfied with his own behavior. The clinician decides to use the Values Assessment to further clarify where values-based action may have the greatest impact. Using the Values Assessment worksheet, Mateo identifies responsibility, family, self-esteem, and health as particularly important to him. He rated his actions as "sometimes" consistent with his values of health and family; and "rarely" consistent with his values of self-esteem and responsibility.

Problem Reframe

Clinician "It seems that in trying to manage your stomach pain, you have felt powerless. You have tried avoiding the distress you feel at work, and using alcohol to help you relax. However, these strategies are causing further conflict and stress. You want to be a good worker, husband, and father, and you feel like you are failing."

Mateo: "Yes, I just feel like a loser."

Treatment

Mateo reports being most misaligned with his values of self-esteem and responsibility. He also expresses feelings of shame and disempowerment. He holds a negative self-concept and expresses his actions are clearly misaligned with his values. Mateo would likely benefit from intervention to contact the responsible and powerful self-perspective of the solar plexus chakra and pursue values-based action towards building strength and self-esteem.

Captain Response-Able

Clinician: "This might sound a little silly, but I would like to try an exercise that might help us gain a different perspective. Are you familiar with any superheroes? Do you have a favorite?"

Mateo: "Yeah, I know a few. I always thought Batman was sort of cool."

Clinician: "Great. I would like you to think a little bit about what makes a superhero. Imagine that you are a superhero. What qualities would you have?"

Mateo: "Well, superheroes are usually brave, strong, and have some kind of moral code or sense of right and wrong."

Clinician: "Mhm, and what do they do when faced with a challenge?"

Mateo: "Save the day?"

Clinician: "Sometimes, yeah. It might not always work out, but a superhero always tries to do something, right?"

Mateo: "Yeah, that's true."

Clinician: "Sometimes we feel powerless and like we cannot do anything. However, like a superhero, we have the power to try. The word 'responsible' means capable of a response. We might not always be successful, but in doing *something* we are using our power to respond."

Mateo: "Hm... I often feel like there is nothing I can do, or that anything I do will not help, so I just don't bother."

Clinician: "When your mind tells you that there is nothing you can do, it makes sense why you would feel stuck. I wonder if it would help to come up with some way of reminding yourself about your superpower to respond, especially when your mind tells you that you are powerless."

Mateo: "Yeah, I need something to help me feel stronger."

Clinician: "Think again about what it might be like to be a superhero. What does a superhero do when they are getting ready for action?"

Mateo: "They might have to put on their super-suit, I suppose."

Clinician: "Sure! Can you think of some small way that you could put on your 'super-suit' when you are needing to prepare for action?"

Mateo: [laughs] "I guess I could imagine zipping up my hero boots. That way I am ready to move and beat-up some bad guys!"

Clinician: "Great! Do you think you might be able to imagine zipping up your hero boots when you are feeling stuck as a reminder that you have the power to take action?"

Mateo: "Sure, I can definitely give it a try."

Building Assertiveness

Clinician: "It seems like it might be helpful for us to talk about your conflict with your co-worker. The way he speaks to you is inappropriate and hurtful. What have you tried so far to address this issue?"

Mateo: "Not much really. I am embarrassed to bring it up. He seems to think he is being funny, and I don't want to be the guy that cannot take a joke. Plus my stomach hurts more whenever I think about talking to my supervisor about it."

Clinician: "I can understand your discomfort, but what has happened as a result of not bringing it up?"

Mateo: "Nothing. It continues to be a problem, and I dread going into work."

Clinician: "How workable is this for you?"

Mateo: "It's really not. I cannot keep going like this."

Clinician: "It can be really difficult to stand up for ourselves and be assertive. It sounds like trying to avoid some of this discomfort in the short-term though has produced problematic longer-term consequences."

Mateo: "Yeah, I know I need to just get over it and do something about it."

Clinician: "Maybe it would be helpful for us to practice together. There is an acronym that explains how to use assertive communication. We say assertive communication is HARD, which stands for honest, appropriate, respectful, and direct. When you talk to your supervisor, I would like you to try this style of communication. Can you think of an example of what you might say?"

Mateo: "Hm. I guess I would like to say that I feel uncomfortable with how this guy makes jokes and speaks about me in front of everyone else. I would like my supervisor to ask him to stop."

Clinician: "Great, how might you say that directly while being honest, appropriate, and respectful?"

Mateo: "Uhm. Hey, Kevin, I wondered if we could talk. I have been feeling uncomfortable with the comments Joe makes about my culture. He also puts me down in front of the team, and it makes it hard for me to come to work sometimes. I am not sure what to do, but I would appreciate your advice and help."

Clinician: "That sounds pretty good! How likely do you think you are to try speaking with your supervisor this week?"

Mateo: "Yeah, I can do that. I think it's time."

Both of these interventions help Mateo tap into his personal power so that he can move his life in the desired direction.

Case #3: Dorothy

Dorothy is a 72-year-old White female. She presents with chronic lower back and hip pain, and does not understand why her primary care provider encouraged her to see a psychologist.

Assessment

Contextual Interview: Dorothy currently lives independently. Three years ago, her husband of 45 years had an affair and ended their marriage. She reported she and her ex-husband did not have a great relationship, but she tried to be a "good wife." She blames herself for the divorce, saying she was too "controlling" and had no interest in physical intimacy. Her ex-husband was the only man she has ever dated, and she is not interested in meeting new people. She states, "Who would want to be with a broken old lady?" She has two adult daughters and six grandchildren. She tries to visit both daughters at least weekly, and calls them once each day. Lately she has been feeling like a burden, and that they do not want to spend time with her. She has one close friend that she talks on the phone with weekly. Dorothy used to be involved in her church community but stopped attending after her divorce. She reports feeling embarrassed, and withdrew from most of her relationships at the time. She was a stay-at-home mother while raising her daughters, and then worked various part-time jobs in retail for several years before retiring. When asked what she does for fun or relaxation, Dorothy states, "Not much, I try to stay busy helping my kids and grandkids" She spends most of her time watching television, and taking care of her home. Her sleep has been poor for several years. She worries at night and has difficulty turning her mind off. She tends to think about past regrets and events she wishes had gone differently. She also worries about her children and grandchildren. They are all doing well, but she "cannot help but worry." She has noticed that her worry seems to annoy her daughters, who often tell her that she needs to "relax." She eats breakfast and dinner most days, and has a small appetite. She tries to go for a walk when the weather is nice. She denies any substance use. Dorothy grew up in a conservative Christian family, and raised her children attending church. Since her divorce, she has struggled with her faith but still tries to read her Bible about each week.

Problem Context: Dorothy reports having back and hip pain for several decades. She is not sure exactly when it started. Several years ago, she did some physical therapy, and did not think it helped. Heating pads and hot showers sometimes help. The pain has worsened over the last few years, but medical images do not show any structural damage that would explain her pain. She describes the pain as an 8/10 on "bad days", and states on average the pain is a 5/10. When the pain is worse, she tries to do as little as possible. On her good days she sometimes "overdoes it." Dorothy does not identify any triggers that seem to make her pain worse, and frustratingly describes the pain as "random."

Stress Evaluation: Dorothy is reluctant to speak with a psychologist and does not understand how her stress could be relevant to her symptoms. The psychologist explains the mind-body connection, and reassures Dorothy that she does not have to talk about anything she is not comfortable with. The psychologist explains that many stressful early life experiences increase the risk of health problems in adulthood, and that it would be helpful to know if she has any of these risk factors. Dorothy agrees to complete the ACE questionnaire. Her ACE score is 6. Prior to age 18, she endorses experiencing physical and emotional neglect and abuse, including sexual abuse, and domestic violence in the home. She reports that she has commonly neglected her own needs and tends to put others first.

Workability: Dorothy states she mostly tries to distract herself from her symptoms. She likes to focus on her children and grandchildren and tries to "keep busy." Dorothy follows a strict daily routine that helps her feel "prepared" in case her pain worsens. This includes taking over-the-counter pain medication routinely in addition to her prescribed pain medication, and avoiding being on her feet for long periods of time. She tries not to talk about her pain and does not tell her children about her pain, saying, "They will just worry."

Chakra Assessment: The clinician draws upon information gathered in the evaluation to determine where chakra dysfunction is likely occurring. Dorothy's prominent physical symptoms are in her lower back and hips, suggesting the sacral chakra. She also reports feelings of guilt and self-blame, and a tendency to self-sacrifice for others, also indicative of sacral chakra problems. Dorothy appears disconnected from the social, playful, and romantic self-perspectives, and misaligned with values of fun/enjoyment and relationships (sacral and heart chakras). Her worry may suggest imbalance in the root chakra. This dispersion of dysfunctional energy is not uncommon. Intervention at any one of these points could be beneficial, but the majority of her distress appears to stem from the sacral chakra.

Problem Reframe

Clinician: "It sounds like you have devoted much of your life to caring for others. You tend to think about others first, and this has partially helped you cope with pain and feel more in control. However, I am also hearing that focusing so much on other people has made it difficult for you to prioritize your own health and happiness. Specifically, it sounds like it is hard for you to think about your own body and feelings. Am I understanding you?"

Dorothy: "I guess so. I don't know how to put myself first, and I am worried I might start crying and never stop if I dwell on my feelings."

Treatment

Dorothy presents with prominent dysfunction of the sacral chakra. She struggles with emotional and self-acceptance, and her preoccupation with feelings of guilt and regret has caused her to limit activities that bring her a sense of excitement or fun. She may struggle with immediately trying to engage in self-gratifying actions, and benefit from initial interventions to develop somatic and self-awareness. This includes accepting her experience as it is and defusing from her physical pain and negative self-stories.

Ocean Breath

Clinician: "I would like to start with building small habits of checking-in with your body and emotions. It feels more natural for you to think about others, so this might be uncomfortable at first. Just like any other new skill, it will take some practice and patience."

Dorothy: "Okay, what do you have in mind?"

Clinician: "Well, there are several ways we can bring our attention to our body. Some of the most common are through focusing on breath, altering our posture, and muscle relaxation. Are you familiar with any of those?"

Dorothy: "No, but I guess I could focus on my breath."

Clinician: "Okay, great. I am going to teach you a breathing technique that might seem a bit strange. If you feel silly at first, that's okay. Sometimes feeling a bit silly helps us see our problems differently. We will start just by taking a few slow, deep breaths. Try to breathe through your nostrils if that is comfortable for you. Practice filling your belly with air as you inhale, and contracting your belly as you exhale. (Practices several diaphragmatic breaths together). How does that feel?"

Dorothy: "Okay, so far."

Clinician: "As we continue, I want you to notice how your body feels and responds to this exercise. If you notice your thoughts drifting away, just gently bring your attention back to your breath. Now, we are going to practice constricting our throat a little so that our breath produces a rushing sound. (Clinician demonstrates Ocean Breath). With each breath, I invite you to picture an ocean wave reaching the shore. (Practice several Ocean Breaths together). What do you notice in your body?"

Dorothy: "This feels weird, but I suppose I feel a bit more relaxed. My mind feels calm."

Clinician: "That's wonderful. The goal of this exercise is to practice observing your breath and physical sensations. If you feel more relaxed, that is a bonus. Sometimes you might notice tension in your body or even pain. That is okay too. We are learning how to observe all of the body's experiences. Do you think you might practice this breathing at home?"

Dorothy: "Yeah, I can try that. Maybe in the mornings would be good."

Room for Regret

Clinician: "You have shared that your mind tends to focus on regrets you have and some of the more painful experiences in your life that you feel guilty about. It sounds like these thoughts deter you from treating yourself with compassion, and giving yourself permission to have more pleasurable experiences."

Dorothy: "I just don't feel like I deserve to put myself first."

Clinician: "I would like to try an exercise that might help us gain a different perspective. There is not a single person whose actions are perfectly aligned with their values all the time. I would like you to think of a specific experience or choice that you feel guilty about. You do not have to share it with me if you do not want to, just hold it in your mind."

Dorothy: "Okay, I have one in my mind."

Clinician: "Alright, now see if you recall what your life was like then. Try to place your awareness behind the eyes of who you were then. Recall the thoughts and feelings you had at the time"

Dorothy: "Ugh. I was dealing with a lot back then."

Clinician: "I can imagine there were painful circumstances. I wonder if this context helps make sense out of why you did what you did."

Dorothy: "Well, yes. I wish things had been different, but I don't know how they could have been."

Clinician: "So it sounds like you did the best you could with the information you had and in the context of your life at the time?"

Dorothy: "I guess that's true."

Clinician: "Do you think it is possible to wish something had happened differently, and still accept the circumstances as they are?"

Dorothy: "I'm not sure...how would that work?"

Clinician: "Well, we start by making room for our disappointment. You might say to yourself, 'I am sad about that experience, and I did the best that I could.' You can be regretful and accepting at the same time."

Dorothy: "That might take some practice."

Clinician: "You are absolutely right. Accepting the things we cannot change does take practice. The next part is reflecting on how we want to move forward. Our pain also highlights for us what we care about most. I am wondering what this regret tells you about what is important to you?"

Dorothy: "Family mostly, and my marriage."

Clinician: "Yeah, you care a lot about your relationships. What do you think your regret then might tell us about what to do in the present?"

Dorothy: "I care about my relationships so much that I think I overwhelm people. I pushed my husband away by trying to take care of everything, and now I am worried I am pushing my daughters away too. I guess I need to listen to my daughters and do more for myself."

Clinician: "That seems like a good place to start. We can start small on building habits of self-care together."

These interventions help Dorothy start to make room for her physical and emotional pain in her awareness. By contacting her pain, she is able to make contact with her values and the part of herself that has been hurting. This will allow her to then start taking action in the direction of her values and self-integration.

Appendices

Appendix A: Evaluation

Contextual Interview

1 Love: *Who do you live with? How is your relationship with each person in the home? What is your relationship status? How long have you been part-nered/married? How are your relationships with family/friends? Who are the most important people in your life?*

2 Work/School: *What do you do for work? Full-time or part-time? Are you in school? Do you enjoy your work/school? How is your work-life balance?*

3 Play: *What do you do for fun or relaxation? Do you have any hobbies? What do you do that is just for you?*

4 Health: *Do you have difficulty falling or staying asleep? How many hours of sleep/night do you get? How is your energy level during the day? Any changes in your diet/appetite? How many meals do you eat? Do you regularly exercise or engage in physical activity? Do you smoke or use other tobacco/nicotine products? How much? Caffeine? Alcohol? Other substances?*

Problem Context

5 Timing: *When did the pain/symptom start? Was anything else significant happening at that time? Was the onset gradual or acute?*

6 Trajectory: *How has the pain/symptom been present over time? Has it been getting progressively worse, fluctuating, or improving? Are there times when the symptom is not present?*

7 Triggers: *What seems to make the pain/symptom worse? Are there any factors that seem to increase the frequency, intensity, or duration of the symptom?*

Stress Evaluation

8 *How much stress have you experienced in your life recently? (0 = none to 10 = severe). Why that number?*

9 *How much stress did you experience as a child? (0 = none to 10 = severe). Why that number?*

10   *How do you cope with or manage stress?*

11   *How would you feel if you discovered that a child you care about was experiencing everything you did as a child?*

Workability Assessment

12   Valued Direction: *What are you seeking? Who and what matters most to you? What direction would you like your life to take? What actions would you like to see yourself doing more, less, or differently that would tell you that you were moving in the "right" direction? What would you do if your pain was no longer a problem for you?* The clinician can also use some variation of the Miracle Question: *If a miracle occurred and you woke up tomorrow and your life was exactly how you would like it to be, what would that look like? What would you be doing? What kind of person would you be? How would you know that you were living your life in a meaningful way?* The purpose of these questions is to understand what the patient would do if they had reduced pain and/or greater function. The patient's answers highlight their values and often naturally translate into functional behavioral goals of treatment.

13   Current Strategies: *What have you tried? What pain management and coping strategies are you currently using? What strategies have you used in the past? What are the "rules" for your pain management?* Listen carefully for avoidance-based strategies. This is also an opportunity to reinforce the patient's problem-solving efforts, validate their distress, and learn from what has not worked.

14   Workability of Strategies: *How are these strategies working for you? Has your pain been reduced? What is or has been the cost of these strategies* (short-term and long-term)*? How are your relationships and activities impacted?*

Appendix B: "FIT" Test

Functional

A. Symptoms begin without physical precipitations (no injury, upon waking in the AM, during times of stress).
B. Symptoms have persisted from an injury that has healed.
C. Symptoms occur in a symmetrical pattern in the body.
D. Symptoms occur on an entire side/half of the body, face, or torso.
E. Symptoms occur in many different body parts at the same time.

Inconsistent

A. Symptoms shift from one location in the body to another.
B. Symptoms are mor ore less intense depending on the time or day of the week.
C. Symptoms occur after, but not during, activity or exercise.
D. Symptoms occur when individual thinks about them or when asked about them.
E. Symptoms occur during periods of increased stress.
F. Symptoms are minimal or non-existent when engaged in joyful or distracting activities.
G. Symptoms are not reliably produced by the same actions.

Triggered

A. Symptoms are triggered by foods, smells, sounds, light, computer screens, menses, changes in the weather, or specific movements.
B. Symptoms are triggered by imagining engaging in a triggering activity.
C. Symptoms are triggered by light touch or mild stimuli, such as the wind or cold.

Created from information presented in Clarke, D. D., Schubiner, H., Clark-Smith, M., & Abbass, A. (Eds.). (2019). Psychophysiologic Disorders: Trauma Informed, Interprofessional Diagnosis and Treatment. Psychophysiologic Disorders Association.

Appendix C: Brief Chakra Assessment

1   Where does the patient primarily experience pain and/or discomfort in their body?
2   What self-perspectives or traits of the patient's self have been lost due to control-based pain management strategies?
3   What painful emotions are prominent?
4   What values have been sacrificed in efforts to control pain?

	Root	Sacral	Solar Plexus	Heart	Throat	Brow
1. Physical Pain	Lower back, feet, ankle, or knee; fatigue, immune condition	Genito-pelvic area hips, bladder, kidney, spleen, reproductive system	Abdomen, stomach/GI tract (e.g., nausea, gastritis), middle spine, pancreas, liver,	Chest, upper back, shoulder, arm, diaphragm or rib area, lungs (dyspnea, hyperventilation, asthma, allergies), accelerated heart rate	Throat, mouth, neck, feelings of choking or difficulty swallowing, esophagitis	Head/face-Migraines, headaches, dizziness, insomnia, sensory dysfunction, sinusitis, seizures
2. Self-Perspectives	Physical & Grounded Active, Family-Oriented, Healthy, Orderly/Organized	Emotional & Playful Adventurous, Funny, Romantic, Sensual	Powerful & Responsible Assertive, Courageous, Independent, Skillful	Compassionate & Social Caring, Generous, Kind, Loving	Honest & Contributing Authentic, Creative, Hard-Working, Humble	Curious & Reflective Imaginative, Insightful, Open-Minded, Wise
3. Emotional Pain	Fear	Guilt, Blame	Anger, Shame	Jealousy, Resentment, Grief	Doubt, Judgment	Depression, Despair
4. Values	Family, Group Belonging, Health, Nature, Physical Activity, Order, Safety, Stability Trust, Self-Care	Adventure, Beauty, Control, Excitement/ Fun, Humor, Pleasure, Romance, Sensuality, Sexuality, Self-Gratification	Assertiveness, Challenge, Courage, Independence, Persistence, Power, Responsibility, Self-Esteem, Skillfulness, Self-Development	Compassion, Empathy, Equality, Forgiveness, Generosity, Intimacy, Kindness, Love, Relationships, Self-Acceptance	Authenticity, Community, Contribution, Creativity, Honesty, Humility, Industry, Justice, Service, Self-Expression	Clarity, Curiosity, Gratitude, Imagination, Knowledge, Mindfulness, Open-Mindedness, Wisdom, Spirituality, Self-Awareness

Appendix D: Circle of Pain Awareness Worksheet

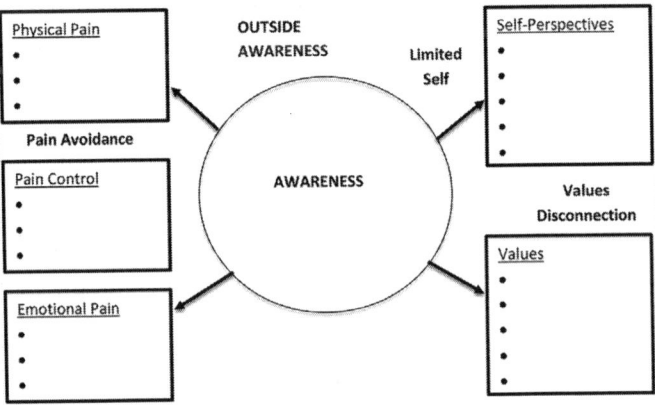

Figure 11.1. Circle of Pain Assessment

1   What are your physical symptoms of pain and/or discomfort? Write in Physical Pain
2   What do you do to manage, control, or avoid your pain/distress? What are the "rules" for keeping physical pain outside the circle? Write in Pain Control
3   What painful emotions are associated with your pain and also get pushed outside the circle? Write in *Emotional Pain* (e.g. fear, guilt, blame, shame, anger, jealousy, resentment, grief, judgment, doubt, depression, despair).
4   What parts of yourself does pain interfere with? Write in *Self-Perspectives* (e.g. active, adventurous, assertive, authentic, caring/compassionate, courageous, creative, family-oriented, funny, generous, grounded, healthy, hard-working, honest, humble, imaginative, independent, insightful, kind, loving, open-minded, orderly/organized, playful, reflective, responsible, romantic, sensual, skillful, social, wise).

5   What values does your pain interfere with? *Write in Values* (e.g. adventure, assertiveness, authenticity, awareness, beauty, challenge, clarity, community service, compassion, contribution, control, courage, creativity, curiosity, empathy, equality, excitement/fun, family, forgiveness, generosity, gratification, gratitude, group belonging, health, honesty, humor, humility, imagination, independence, industry, integrity, intimacy, justice, kindness, knowledge, love, mindfulness, nature, open-mindedness, order, persistence, physical activity, pleasure, power, relationships, responsibility, romance, safety, self-acceptance, self-care, self-development, self-esteem, self-expression, sensuality, sexuality, skillfulness, spirituality, stability, trust, wisdom).

6   What if you have to make room for your pain (physical + emotional) in order to contact what is important to you? We have to make room for the pain on the left side to also make room for the self and values on the right side. What are you willing to make room for? *Experiment with one new thing at a time.*

Appendix E: COACT Skills Assessment

	Rate Skill Level	Examples
Nonattachment (Defusion and Acceptance Skills)	1 = Lacking Skill 2 = Limited Skill 3 = Average Skill 4 = Strong Skill	• Willing to experience pain in order to engage in meaningful activities • Makes room for all emotions, even painful ones • Responds to pain consciously according to values, rather than relying on automatic responses (i.e. rules of pain avoidance) • Views pain as only part of their experience, and is able to observe their pain without entanglement
Somatic Awareness (Present Moment Skills)	1 = Lacking Skill 2 = Limited Skill 3 = Average Skill 4 = Strong Skill	• Flexible attention to sensations in the body • Able to be present with sensations in the body, without trying to alter or change them • Open and curious stance towards physical sensations. • Observes and acknowledges physical sensations as they are (not exaggerating or minimizing).
Self-Integration (Self-as-Context Skills)	1 = Lacking Skill 2 = Limited Skill 3 = Average Skill 4 = Strong Skill	• Makes room for all aspects of the self, even painful parts. • Does not reject parts of self or experience • Flexible self-definition • Able to shift perspectives • Practices self-compassion and kindness • Able to take the perspective of the "true" self, defused from self-stories and emotions

	Rate Skill Level	Examples
Values-Based Action (Values and Committed Action Skills)	1 = Lacking Skill 2 = Limited Skill 3 = Average Skill 4 = Strong Skill	• Actions are clearly tied to values • Does not engage in actions counter to values • Aware of what is important to them • Appropriately pursues values even with some levels of pain

Appendix F: Self-Perspectives Assessment

Read the list of characteristics below and circle the ones that are most important to you. This is not a complete list, and you may write others that come to mind.

1   active, family-oriented, grounded, healthy, orderly/organized
2   adventurous, funny, playful, romantic, sensual
3   assertive, courageous, independent, responsible, skillful
4   caring/compassionate, generous kind, loving, social
5   authentic, creative, hard-working, honest, humble
6   imaginative, insightful, open-minded, reflective, wise

Which traits are most important to you?

Does your experience of pain interfere with your actions fulfilling these traits?

Characteristics/Trait	My actions are consistent with this trait (0 = Never, 1 = Rarely; 2 = Sometimes; 3 = Usually; 4 = Nearly Always)
1.	
2.	
3.	
4.	
5.	
6.	
7.	
8.	
9.	

Appendix G: Values Assessment

Read the list of values below and circle the ones that are most important to you. You may also circle all that are even somewhat important to you, and underline the ones that are especially important. This is not a complete list of all values, so you may write others that come to mind.

1   family, group belonging, health, nature, order, physical activity, safety, self-care, stability, trust
2   adventure, beauty, control, excitement/fun, gratification, humor, pleasure, romance, sensuality, sexuality
3   assertiveness, challenge, courage, independence, persistence, power, responsibility, self-development, self-esteem, skillfulness
4   compassion, empathy, equality, forgiveness, generosity, intimacy, kindness, love, relationships, self-acceptance
5   authenticity, community service, contribution, creativity, honesty, humility, industry, integrity, justice, self-expression
6   awareness, clarity, curiosity, gratitude, imagination, knowledge, mindfulness, open-mindedness, spirituality, wisdom

What does pain stop you from doing? How does pain interfere with your actions fulfilling these values?

Value (Rank Importance)	My actions are consistent with this value (0 = Never, 1 = Rarely; 2 = Sometimes; 3 = Usually; 4 = Nearly Always)
1.	
2.	
3.	
4.	
5.	
6.	
7.	

Appendix H: Somatic Awareness Tracking

Date/Time	Body Part	Sensation	Thought/Feeling	Exercise Practiced?	Observations

Appendix I: Self-Integration Outline

1   Part of my self-story I want to let go of is _____
2   Part of myself or feeling I want to make room for is _____
3   The self I want to contact is _____
4   I can build this connection by doing _____

Appendix J: Committed Action Plan

My Value(s):
Pain Control————————————————————————Values

1   Where are you in reference to behaving according to your values or according to pain control? Is this where you want to be?
2   What value do you want to invest more time in energy towards?
3   What specific goals do you have for this value?
4   What steps can you take towards these goals?
5   How can you track this? When will you do this?
6   What skills or resources do you need to achieve this goal?
7   What barriers might make it difficult for you to achieve this goal? What can you do to cope with these challenges?

Appendix K: Chakra Interventions

Root Chakra Interventions

Nonattachment

- Inhale your experience (take it in) like the smell of a flower or fresh grass. "Hold your experience like a delicate flower in your hand"
- Practice responding flexibly to your pain like a bendy tree
- Imagine placing each painful thought/sensation/emotion on a leaf falling off a tree
- Defuse with Exercise: engage in physical activity (dancing, walking, jumping-jacks)
- Mindful Physical Activity

Somatic Awareness

- Mountain Pose
- Tree Pose
- Cat-Cow
- Head-to-Knee
- Knee-to-Chest
- Downward Facing Dog
- Diaphragmatic Breathing

Self-Integration

- Strong Body
- Thank the Body
- Facing Your Fear
- Inner Safe Space
- You Belong Here

Values-Based Action

- Exercise/Physical Activity
- Values-Based Activity Pacing

- Enjoy the Outdoors
- Self-Care
- Family/Cultural Engagement
- Build Your Safe Space

Sacral Chakra Interventions

Nonattachment

- Savor your experience like a bite of your favorite dessert. "Take in your experience like a drink of pure water"
- Practice responding flexibly to your pain like an ocean wave
- Imagine placing each painful thought/sensation/emotion on a wave crashing on the beach
- Laughter is the Best Medicine: think of a funny memory
- Mindful Play

Somatic Awareness

- Hip Circles
- Pelvic Rock
- Forward Bend
- Half Sun Salutation
- Butterfly
- Open Angle
- Goddess Pose
- Ocean Breath

Self-Integration

- Laugh at Yourself
- Let's Play
- Embracing Emotions
- Room for Regret
- Alignments

Values-Based Action

- Play!
- Healthy Pleasures
- Choose Your Adventure
- Silliness is the Spice of Life
- Make Time for Romance
- Treat Yourself

Solar Plexus Chakra Interventions

Nonattachment

- Observe your experience like the flickering flames of a birthday candle. Witness your experiences like a roaring bonfire.
- Practice responding flexibly to your pain like a dancing flame
- Imagine placing each painful thought/sensation/emotion on a piece of ash floating out of a fire
- Powerful Disobedience: say or think one thing and do another, or intentionally create a false thought
- Mindful Eating

Somatic Awareness

- Seated Twist
- Elbow-to-Knee Twist
- Seated Side Angle
- Revolved Abdomen
- Boat Pose
- Bow Pose
- Bird Dog
- Bellows Breath

Self-Integration

- Captain Response-Able
- Just Trying to Help
- Choose Your Character
- Facing the Bully
- Anger Shield

Values-Based Action

- Responsible Action
- Strength Building
- Go Your Own Way
- Master It
- "Just Because I Choose To"
- Building Assertiveness

Heart Chakra Interventions

Nonattachment

- Hold your experience like a soft pillow. "Embrace your experience like a crying child." "Inhale your experience like a deep breath"

- Practice responding flexibly to your pain like a gust of wind
- Imagine placing each painful thought/sensation/emotion on clouds in the sky
- Defusing Breath: focus on your breath and think, "here, now" as you inhale and exhale
- Mindful Breathing

Somatic Awareness

- Arm Movements: Arm Circles, Vertical/Horizontal Arm Raises, Serving Arms
- Crossed Hug
- Half Wheel
- Bridge
- Cobra
- Upward Facing Dog
- Sighing Breath

Self-Integration

- Heart-to-Heart
- Puppy Love
- Bigger or Bitter?
- Enough for Everyone
- Love & Loss

Values-Based Action

- Social Engagement
- Self-Compassion
- Forgiveness
- Intimacy
- Grieving with Love

Throat Chakra Interventions

Nonattachment

- Sing to your experience like you a sleeping child. Listen to your experience like you would a dear friend.
- Practice responding flexibly to your pain like a musical note or reverberating sound
- Imagine placing each painful thought/sensation/emotion on musical notes or the signs of soldiers on parade

- Sing It/Silly Voice: Sing the painful thought to the tune of a familiar song or say it in a silly/cartoon voice
- Mindfulness with Words

Somatic Awareness

- Neck Stretches
- Chin Tucking
- Fish Pose
- Lion's Breath
- Bumblebee Breath

Self-Integration

- Court Stenographer
- The Overheard Conversation
- Vocal Warm-Ups/Vocal Awareness
- Where do you Give?
- 80th Birthday

Values-Based Action

- Sound of Silence
- Learn to Listen
- Where Did You Hear That?
- Make Your Mark
- Creative Expression
- Conscious Intentions

Brow Chakra Interventions

Nonattachment

- Look at your experience like an artistic masterpiece. Internalize your experience like the wisdom of a master.
- Practice responding flexibly to your pain like bouncing light
- Imagine placing each painful thought/sensation/emotion on lightning bolts or send them across a rainbow
- Name It, Describe It, and Thank It: defuse from pain by externalizing it. Describe your pain by name or physicalize it's features (e.g. color, size, shape, form, texture, etc.). Thank your pain/body/mind for trying to help keep you safe.
- Mindfulness with Imagery

Somatic Awareness

- Savasana
- Easy Pose
- Child's Pose
- Pigeon
- Alternate Nostril Breathing

Self-Integration

- Sitting with Sadness
- Different Glasses
- The You Behind It All
- General Perspective Taking: Words of Wisdom, Movie/Book Metaphor, What Could This Be?

Values-Based Action

- Open Mind
- Meditation/Mindfulness
- Journaling
- Spiritual Practice
- Gratitude
- Perspective-Taking

Index

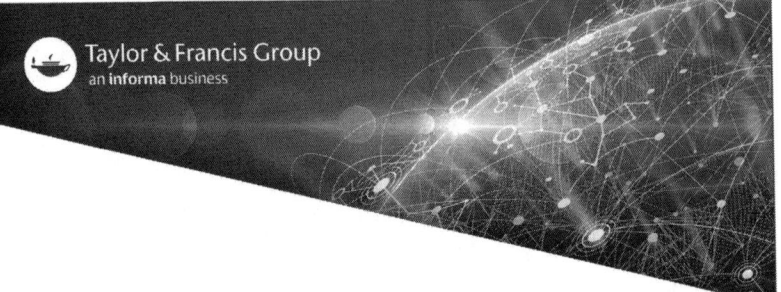
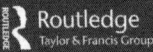
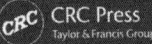